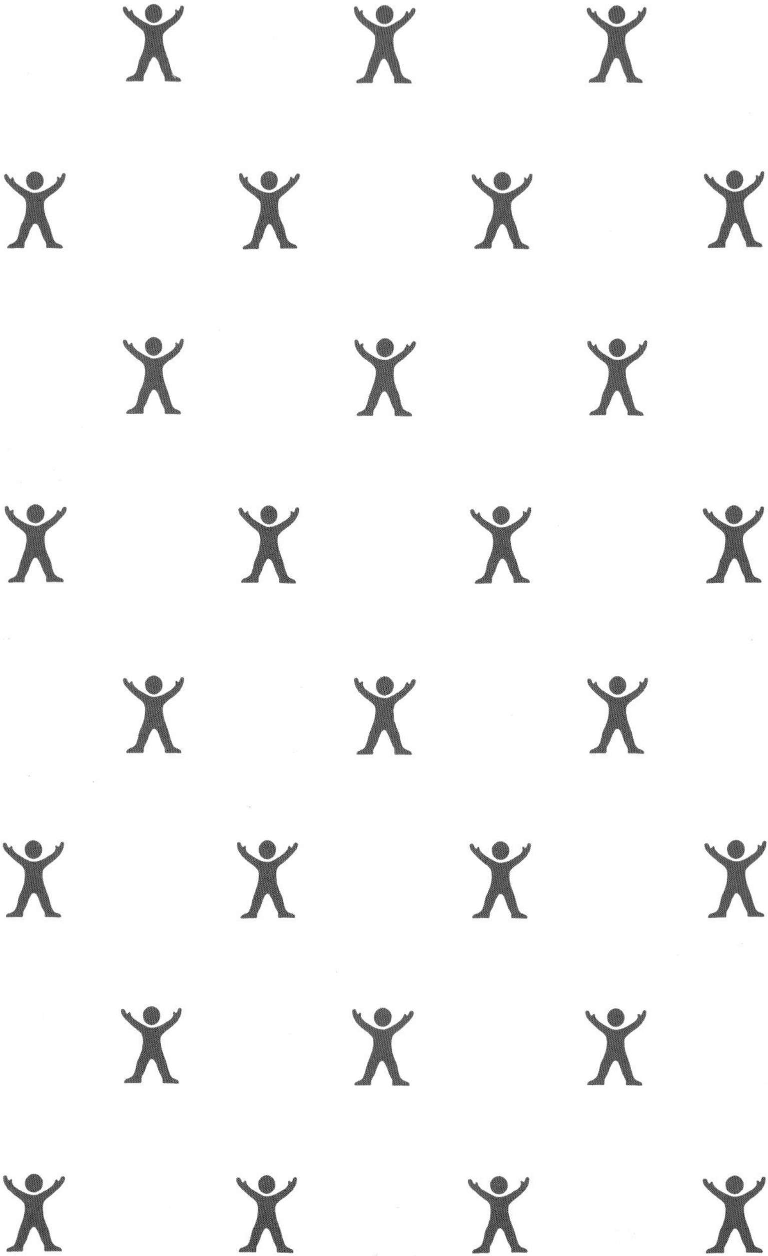

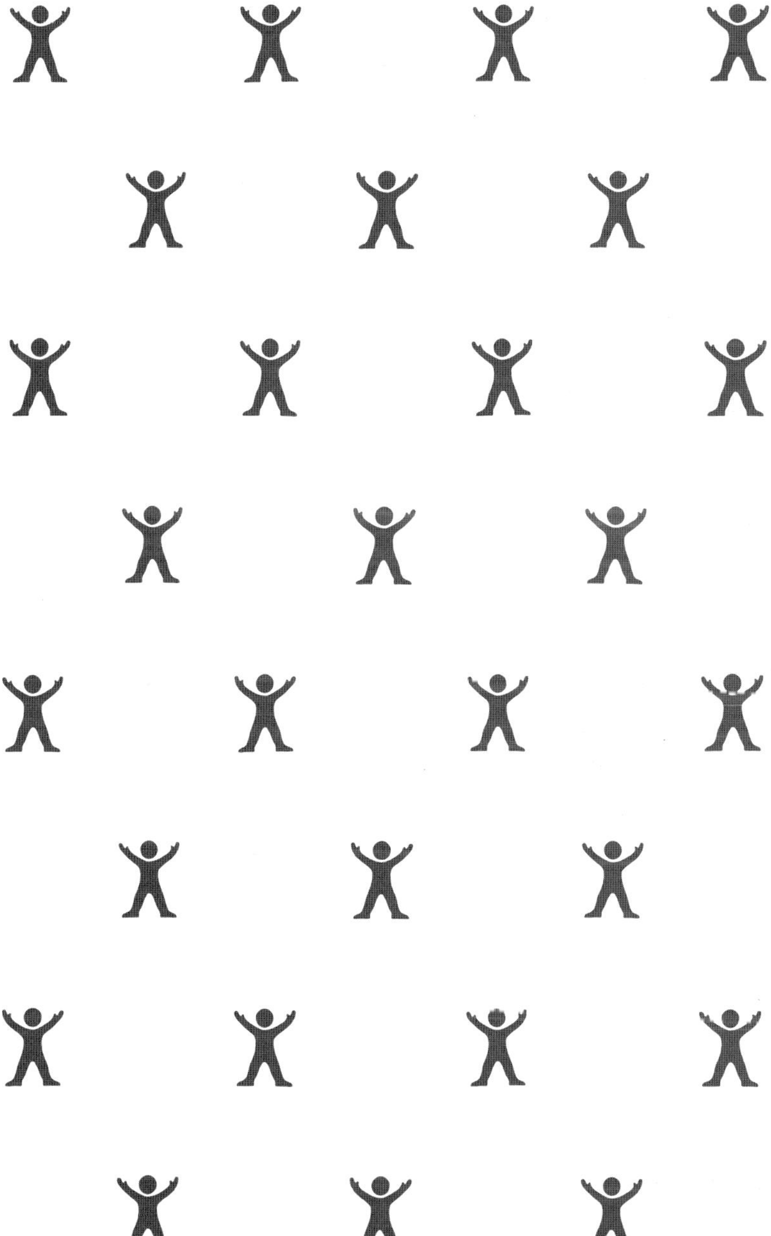

KINGFISHER
Kingfisher Publications Plc
New Penderel House
283–288 High Holborn
London WC1V 7HZ

Originally published in hardback by Kingfisher 1993
under the series title *Young World*
This edition published in 1999

2 4 6 8 10 9 7 5 3 1

1TR / 0299 / EDK / (MAR) / 135MA

A CIP catalogue record for this book
is available from the British Library.

ISBN 0 7534 0380 3

Printed in Spain

FIRST FACTS

My Body

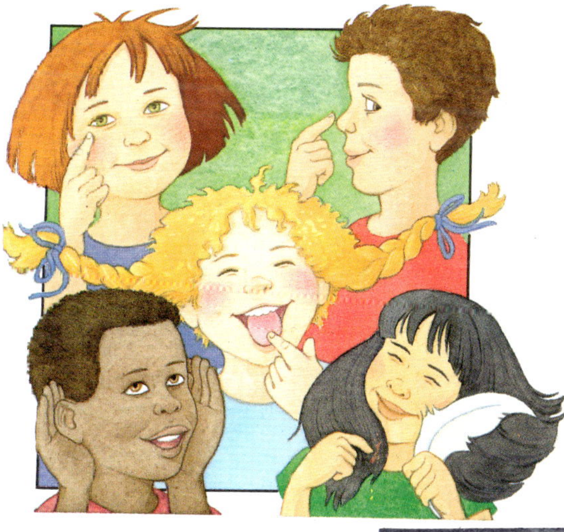

KINGfISHER

Authors
Florence and Pierre-Olivier Wessels

Medical adviser
Dr Jean-Baptiste Carlander

Translator
Patricia Crampton

Series consultant
Brian Williams

Editor
Véronique Herbold

Designers
Gérard Finel and Martine Pfeiffer

Illustrators
Denise Bazin
Danièle Schulthess
Michèle Trumel

About this book

Every minute of the day, our bodies are busy working – while we wash and dress and eat, while we play and sleep. Different parts of the body work together to let us see, move and grow. How does this happen? What do the parts we can't see look like?

This book shows you how the human body works. It is arranged in sections, so you can read about the parts of the body (such as the brain and bones), the systems (such as the heart), and the senses (such as eyesight and hearing). It describes how babies grow into children and children into adults, and how we can look after our bodies sensibly. The human body is amazing, and this book is full of amazing information about it.

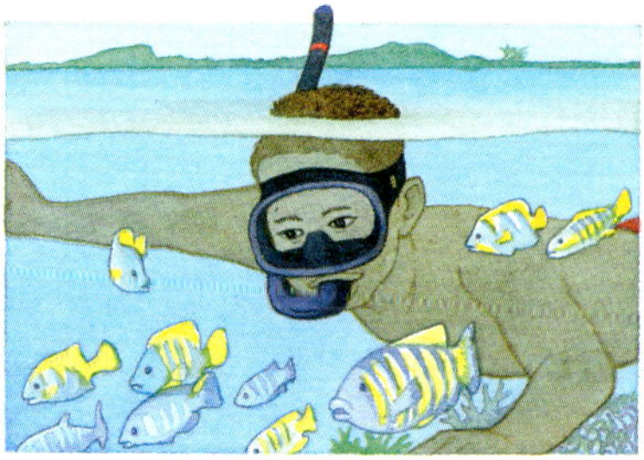

CONTENTS

MY BODY

FROM HEAD TO FOOT

LIFE STORY

THE SENSES

THE SYSTEMS

KEEPING FIT

My body

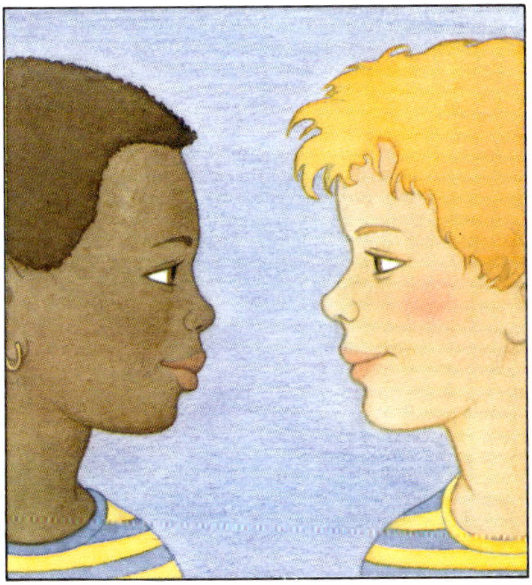

One person, one body

There are five billion human beings on Earth. We all have a body made to the same design.

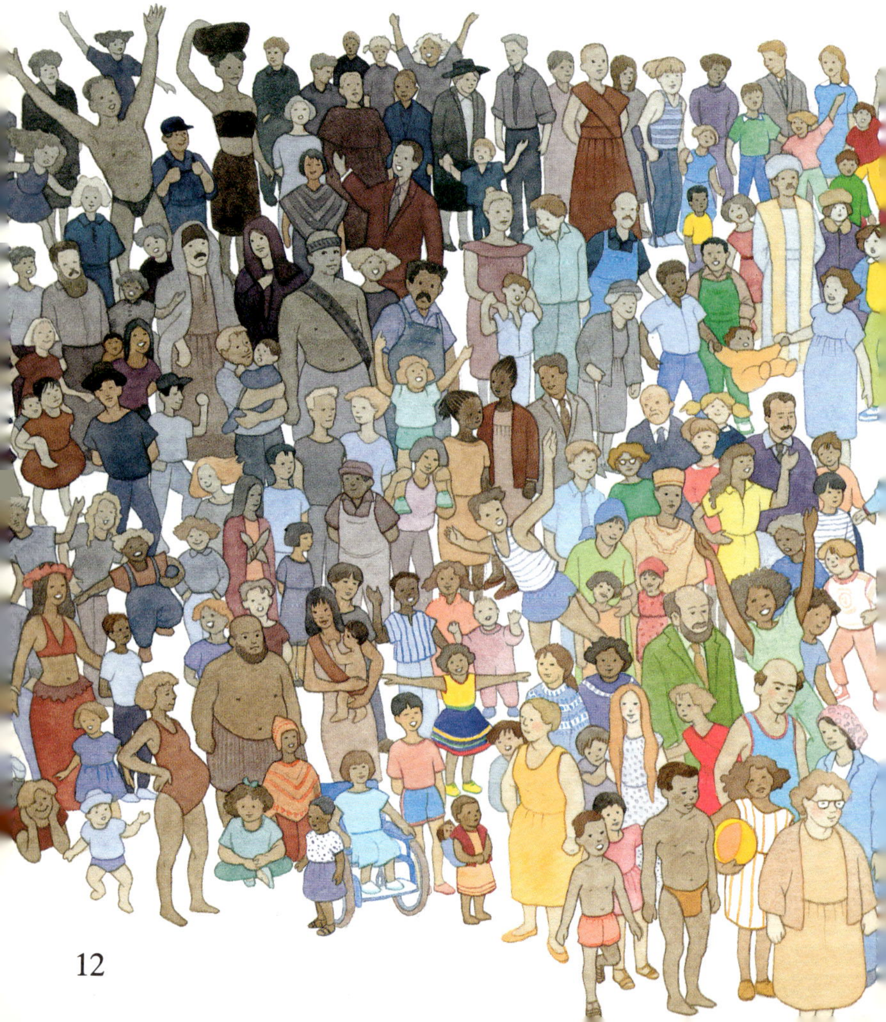

Human bodies are alike, but at the same time everyone is different! No one else is the same as you. You are unique.

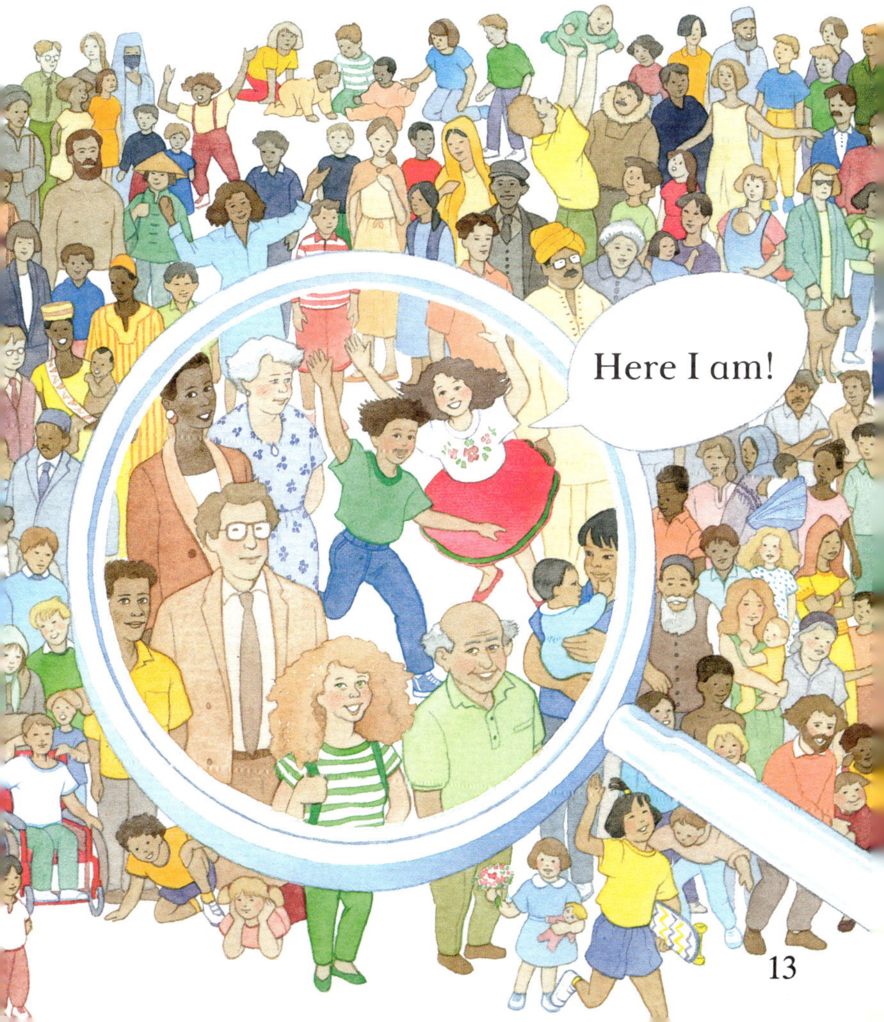

Differences

Children and adults, girls and boys, tall people and short people – we are all human beings, but we are all different.

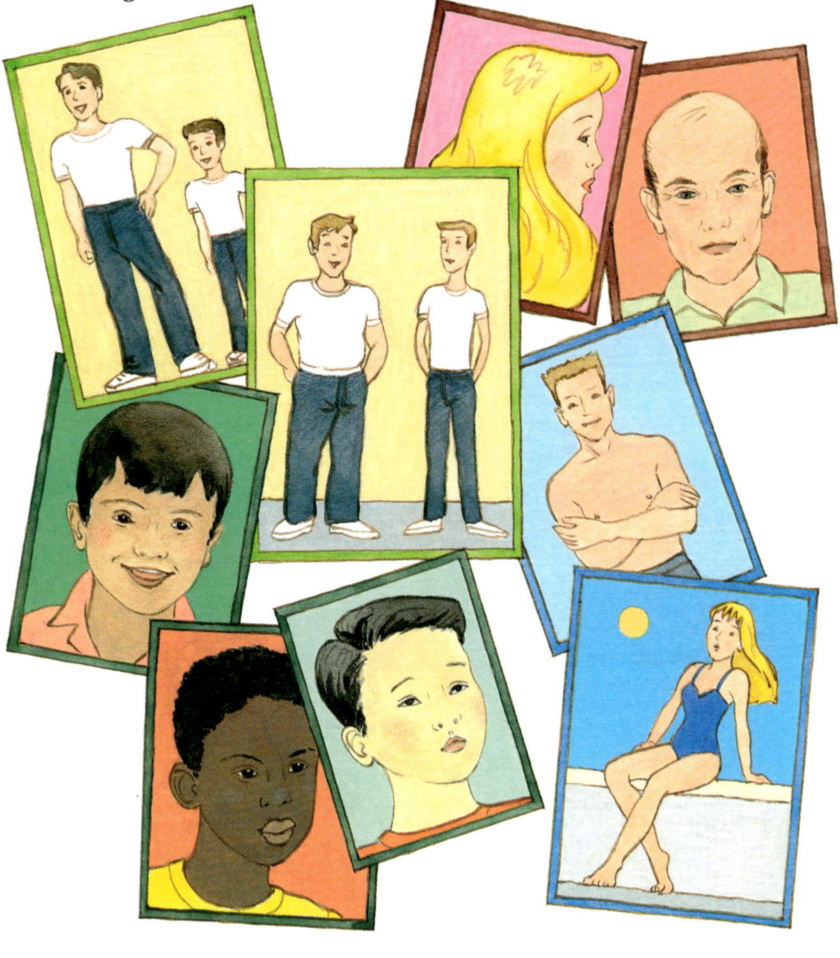

Lots of details make us different from one another. The colour of our hair and skin... the shape of our eyes, ears, lips, nose, and chin... the way we stand, walk and talk.

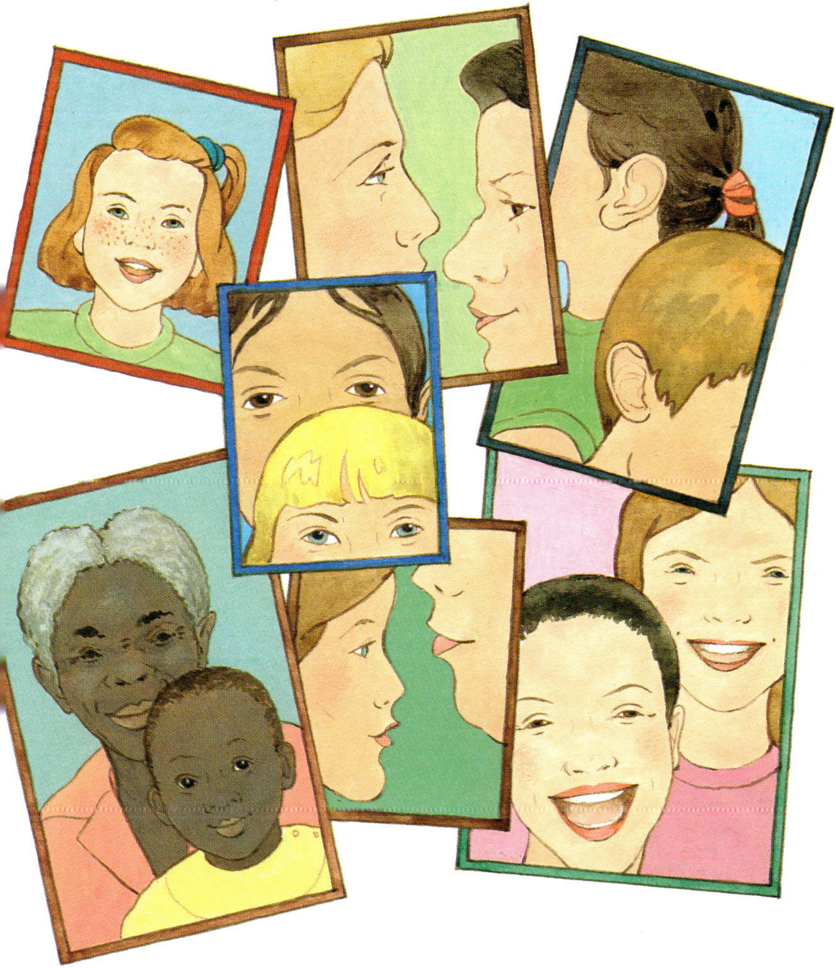

Likenesses

People who belong to the same family often look similar. Brothers and sisters are alike, and children resemble their parents.

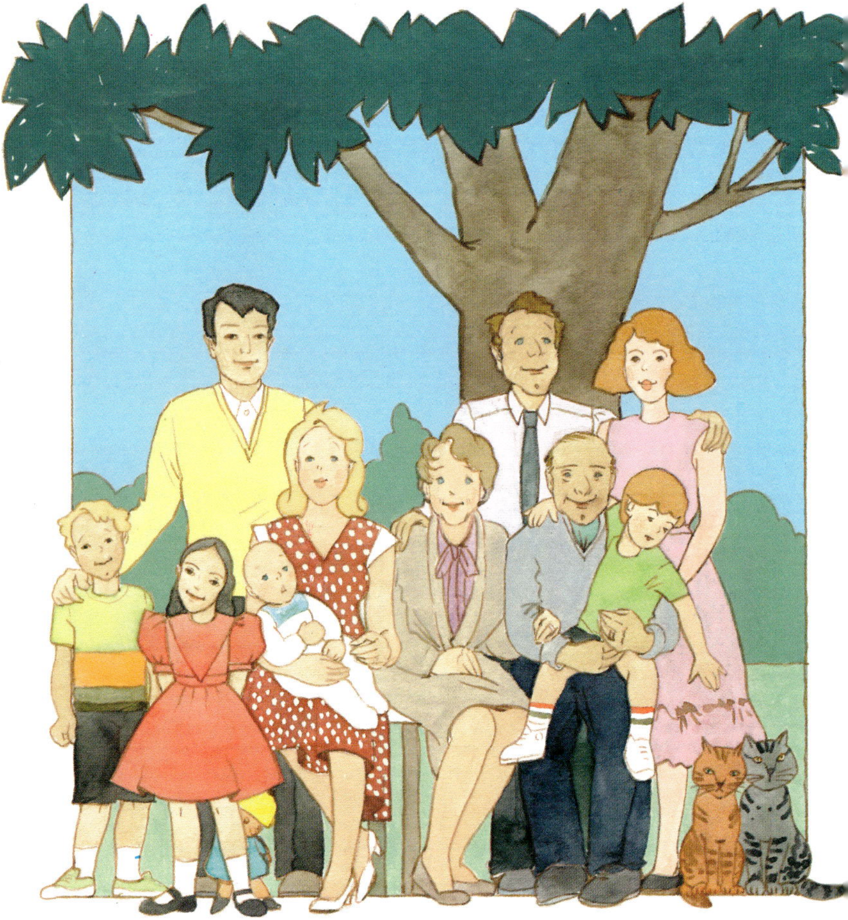

Twin brothers and twin sisters can look almost exactly alike. You have to get really close to them to find out who is who.

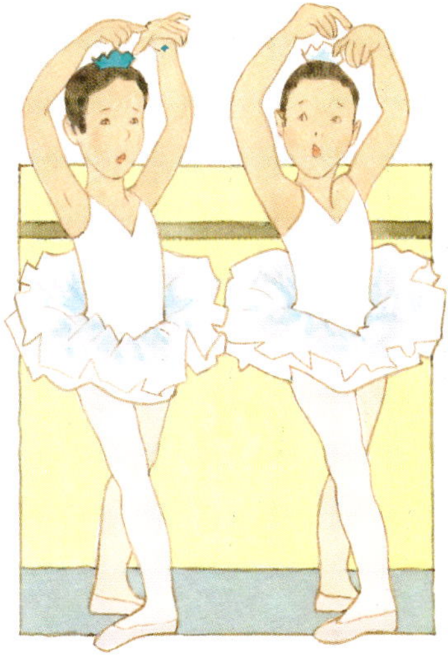

This family tree shows three generations of one family:

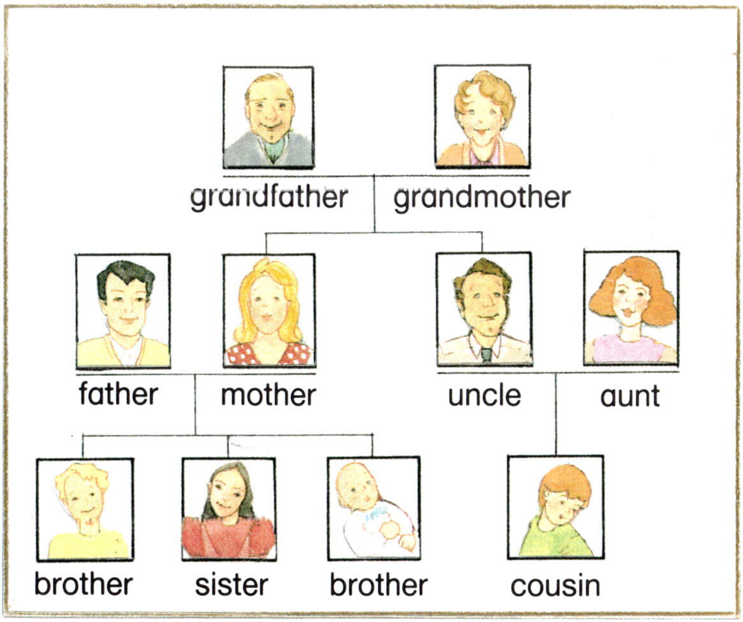

A body for living

The body is like a clever machine that can do lots of things. It can laugh, cry, talk, walk, run and jump.

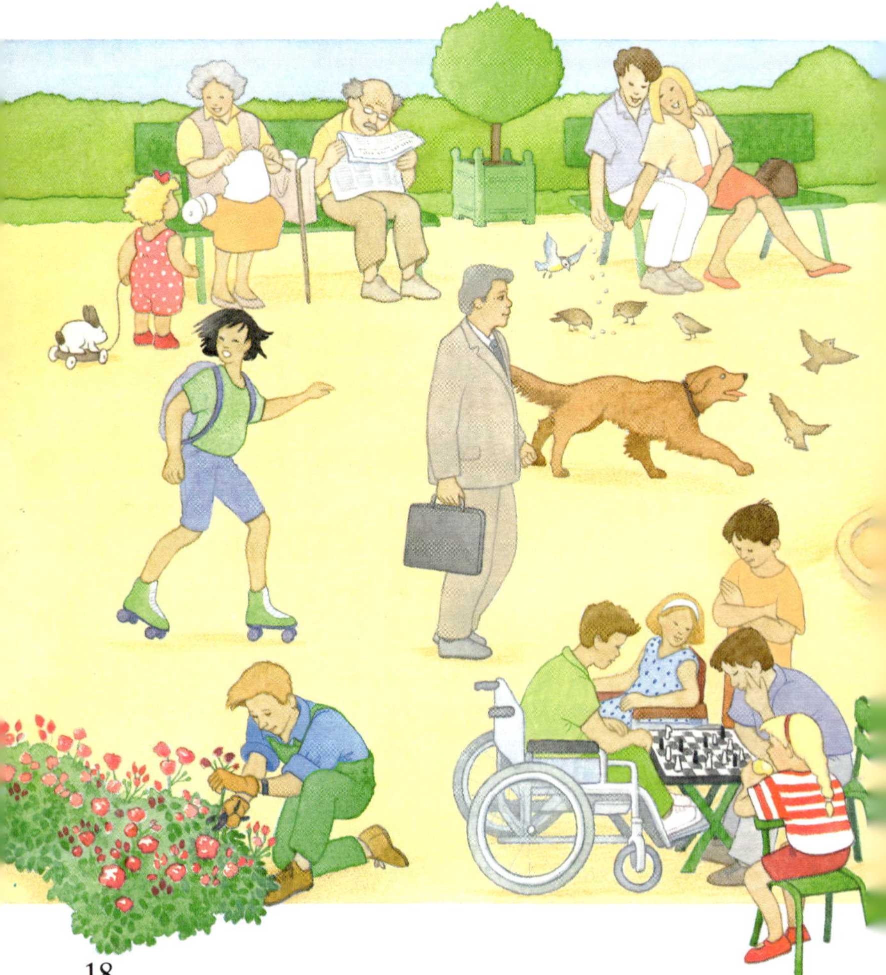

The body can also read, think, love, play, work and rest.

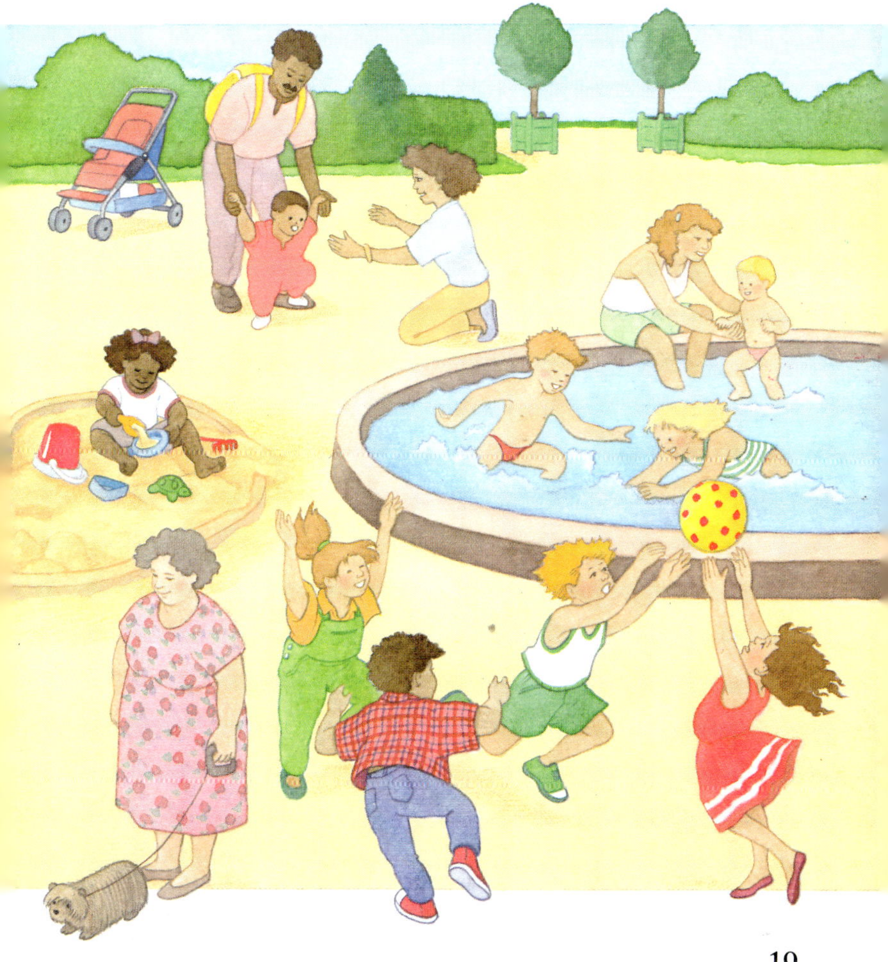

A body for everywhere

People want to go every-where, and they can.

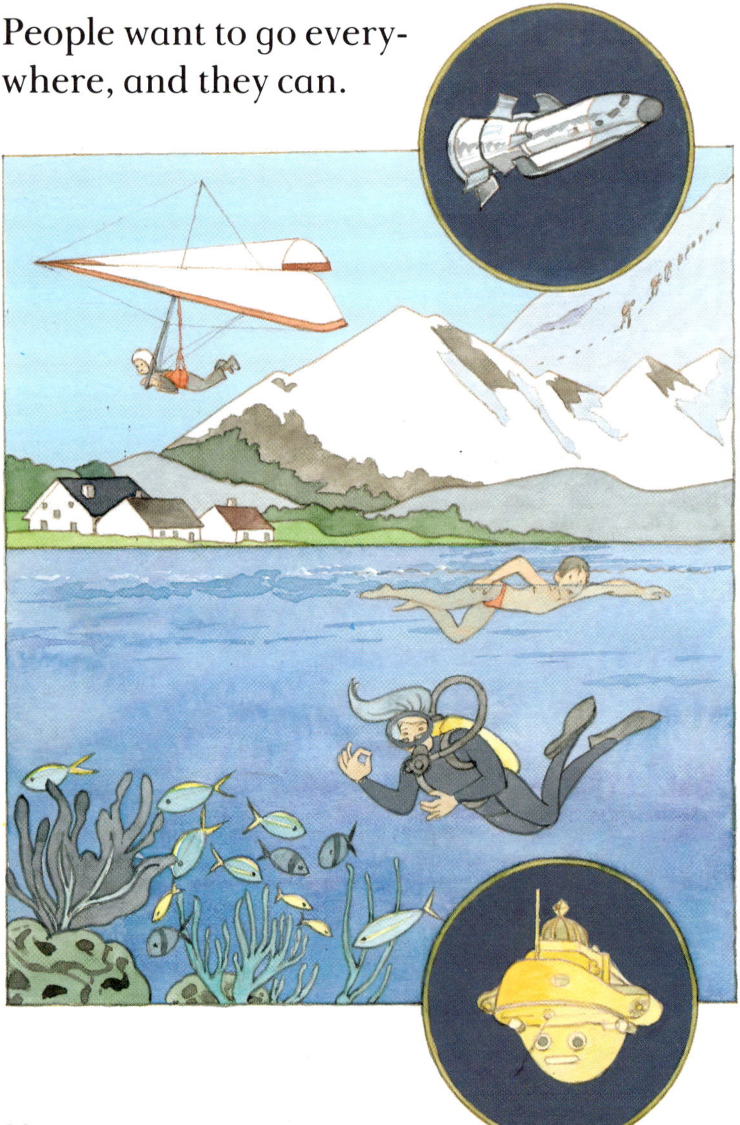

People can travel high in the sky, explore Space, and dive down through the ocean.

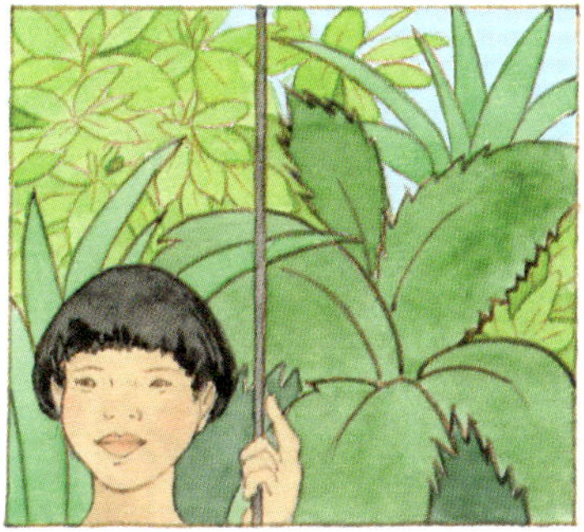

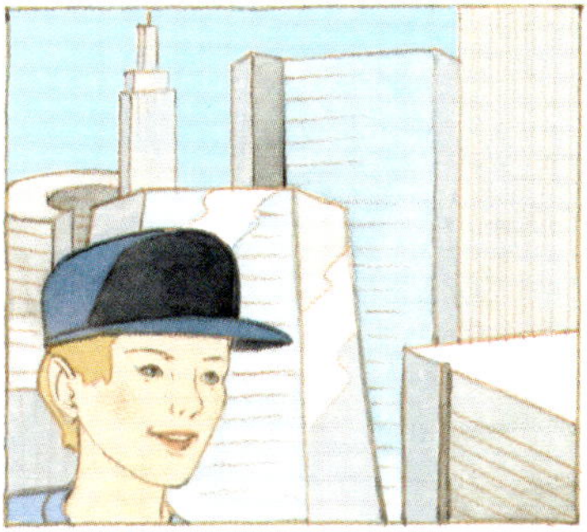

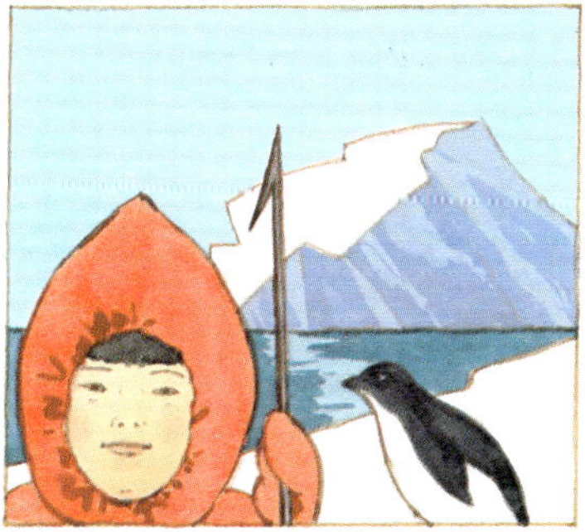

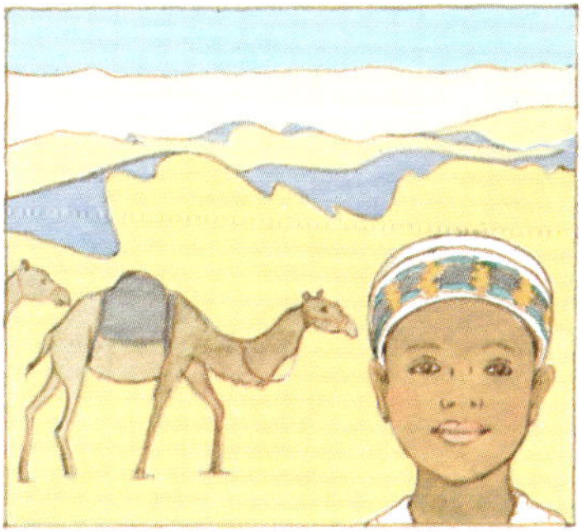

People live in rainforests and towns, in frozen lands and hot deserts. The human body has adapted or changed to live in different conditions.

The history of the body

The story of the human body began three and a half million years ago.

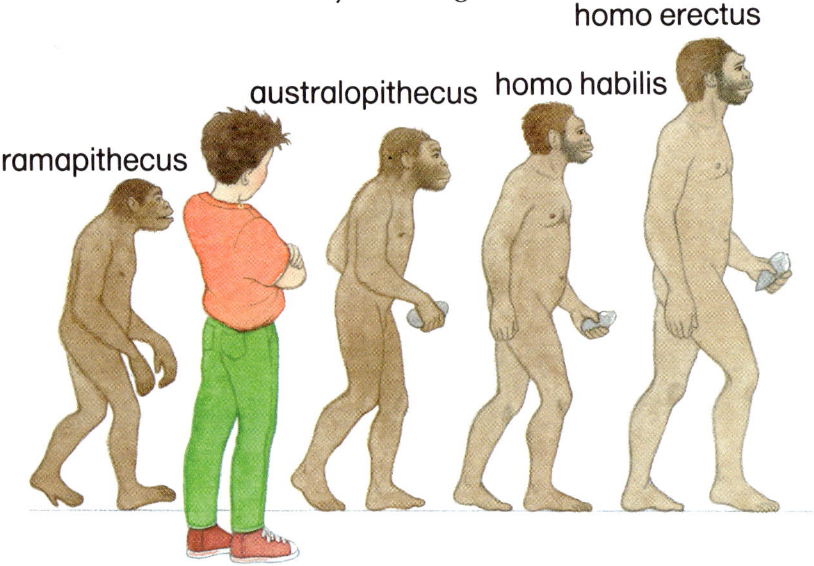

Since then, the human body has changed.

Scientists find bones of people who lived long ago, and study the differences between their bodies and ours.

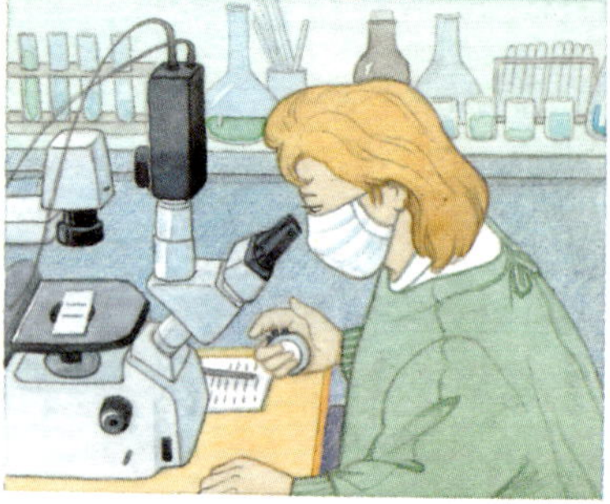

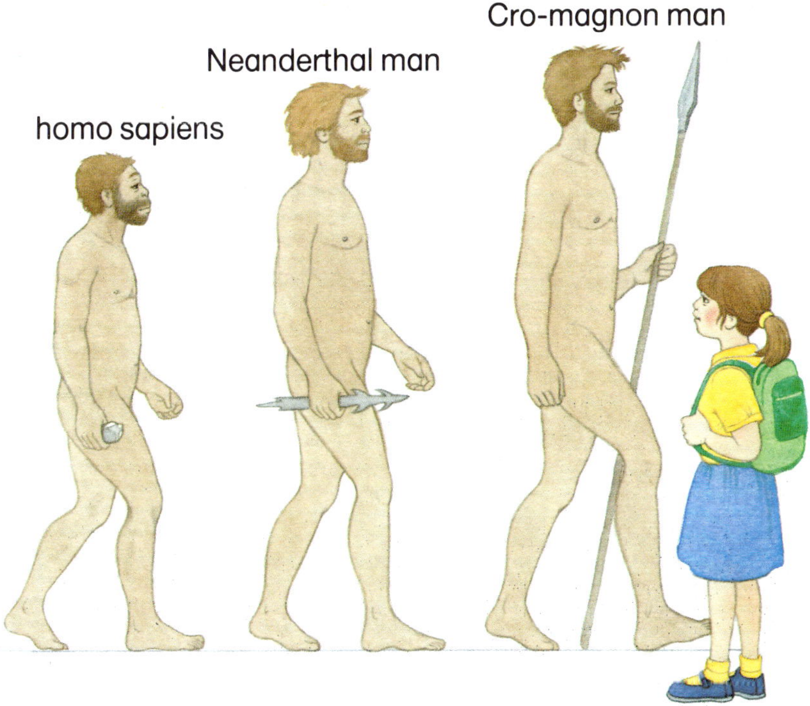

The change from the first humans to ourselves is called evolution.

Nowadays an eight-year-old child is as tall as an adult australopithecus. She knows much more than the first humans knew. She lives three or four times longer. This is because she lives in better conditions.

Amazing facts

- Like cats and whales, human beings are mammals. All mammal mothers make milk in their bodies to feed their babies.

- A double is someone who looks exactly like another person, without being his or her twin.

- The science which studies the similarities between parents and their children is called genetics.

- The first true human beings lived about two million years ago, in Africa. Scientists call this type homo habilis.

From head

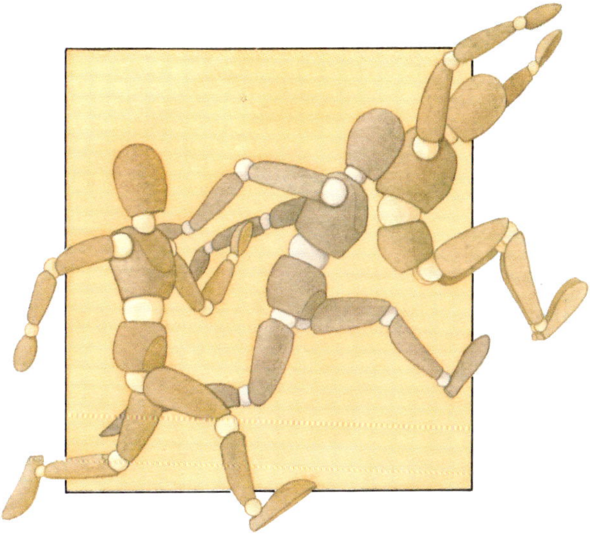

to foot

Body parts

The human body has a head, a torso, two upper limbs which are our arms, and two lower limbs which are our legs.

These parts of the body help it to do different things.

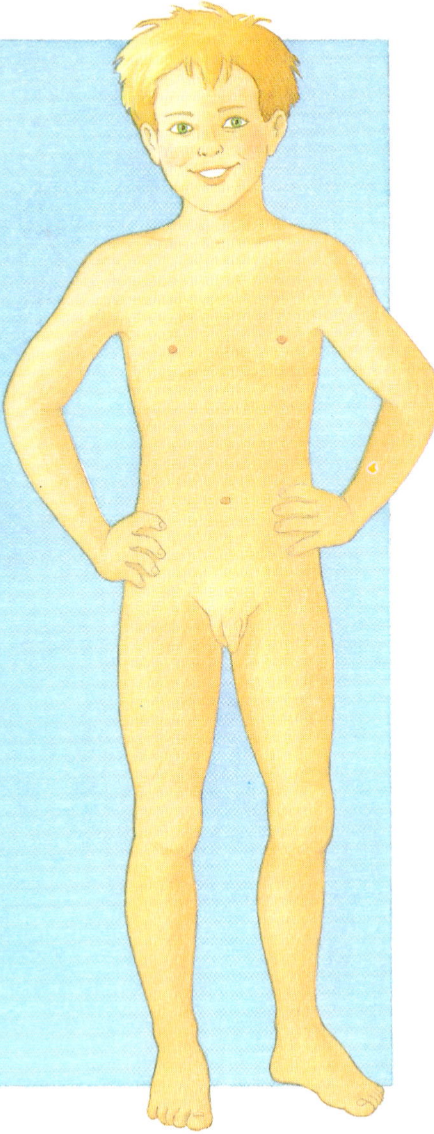

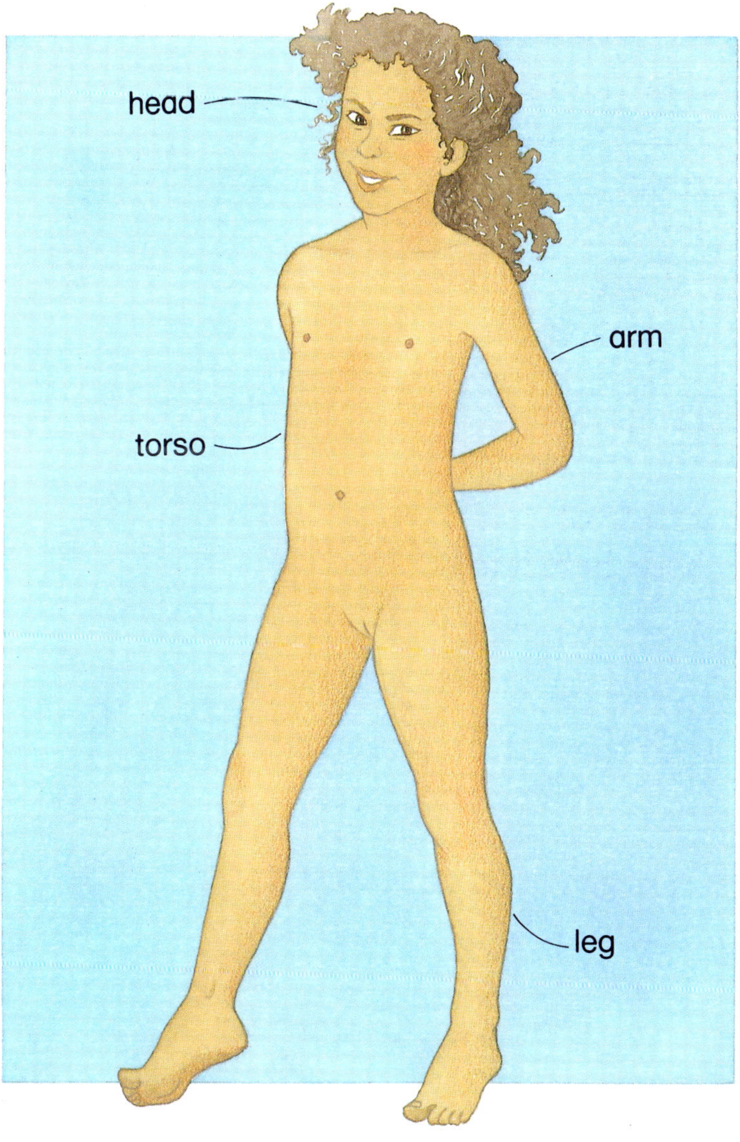
head
arm
torso
leg

The skin

Skin covers the whole body.

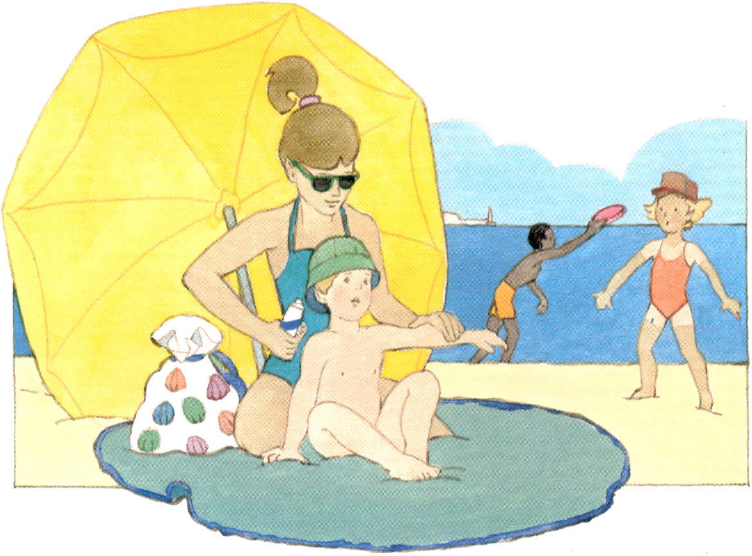

Skin keeps the parts inside us safe.

Skin is very sensitive to the sun's rays and may get burned. Suncream protects it.

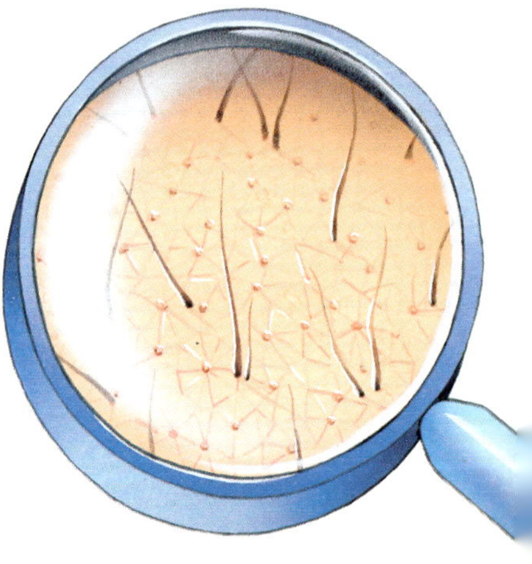

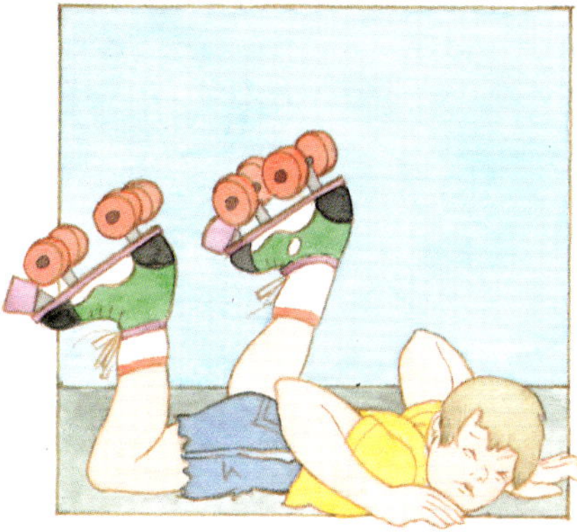

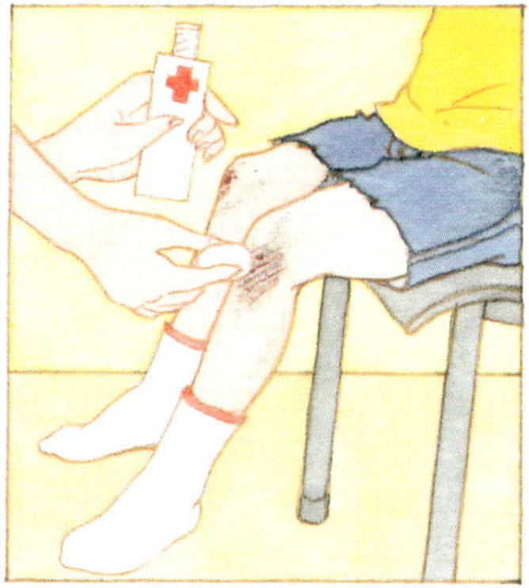

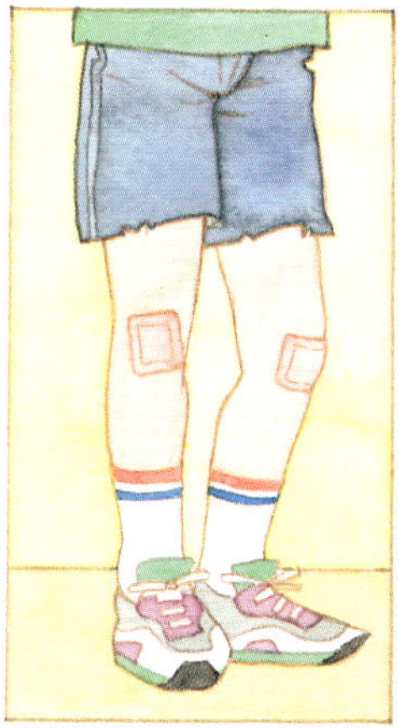

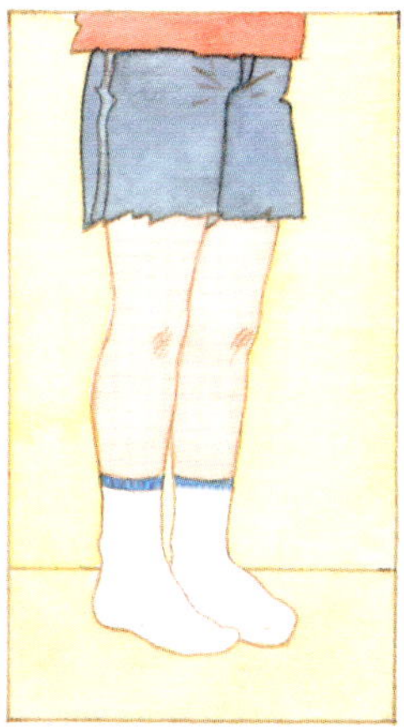

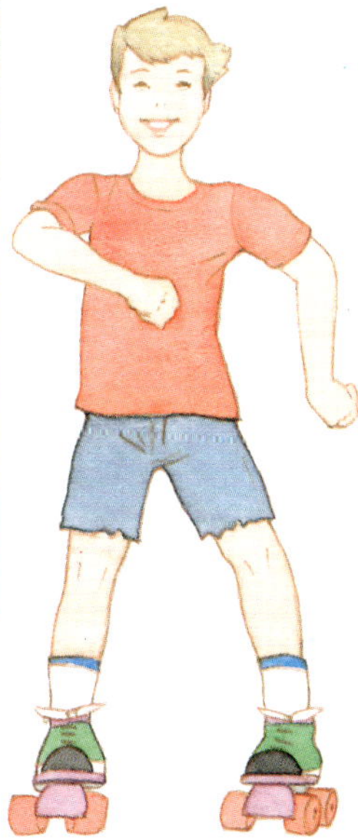

Grazed skin bleeds.
The wound must be cleaned,
to get rid of dirt and germs.
A bandage keeps the wound clean and dry.
The blood dries and forms a scab. New skin
grows under the scab, and the scab falls off.

Marks on the skin

Skin has pigments or colouring called melanin. Melanin helps protect the skin from sunlight. Freckles often appear on fair skin that has been in the sun. They are patches of extra melanin.

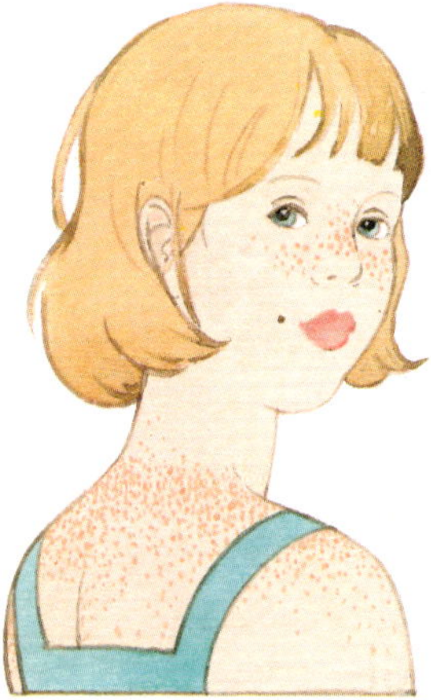

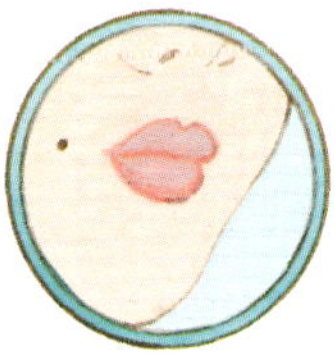

Moles are permanent patches of melanin.

Sometimes our faces change colour! People turn red with embarrassment, and white with shock.

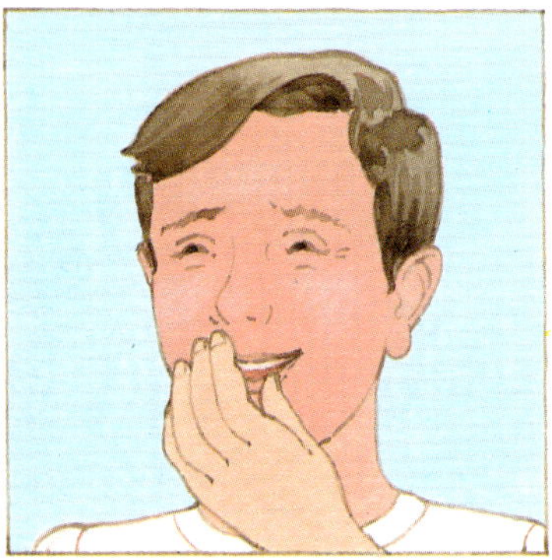

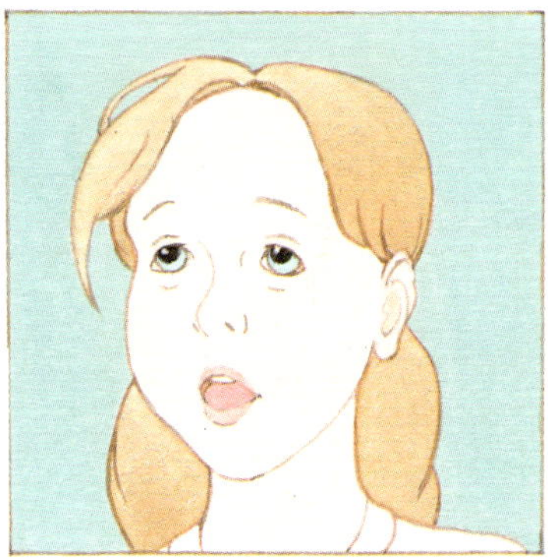

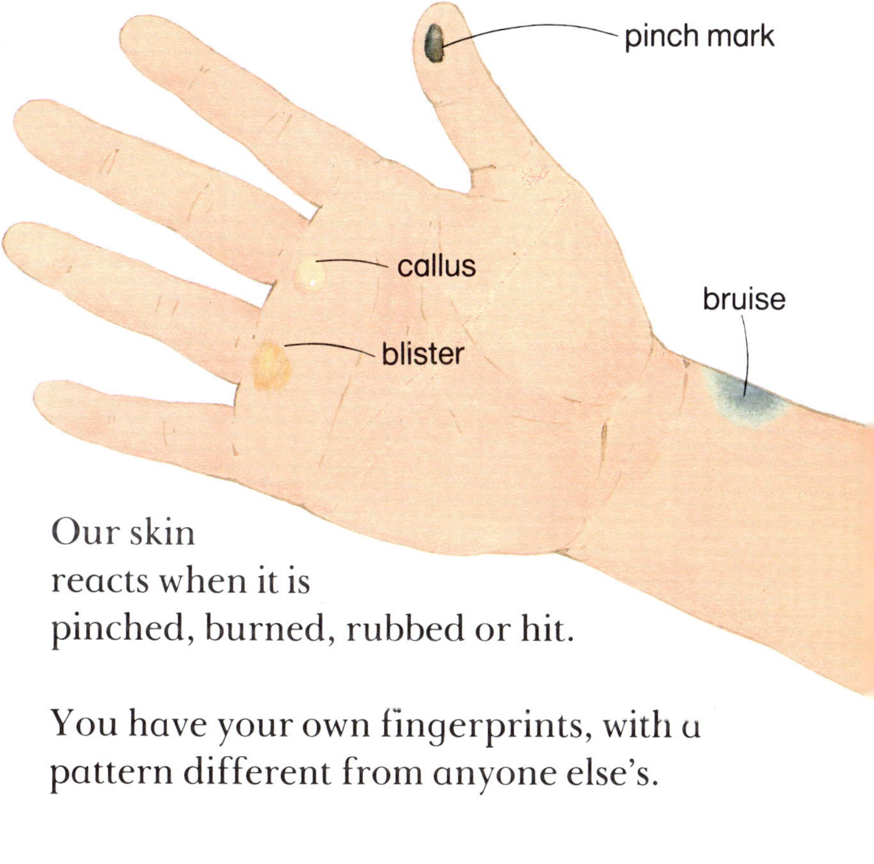

Our skin
reacts when it is
pinched, burned, rubbed or hit.

You have your own fingerprints, with a
pattern different from anyone else's.

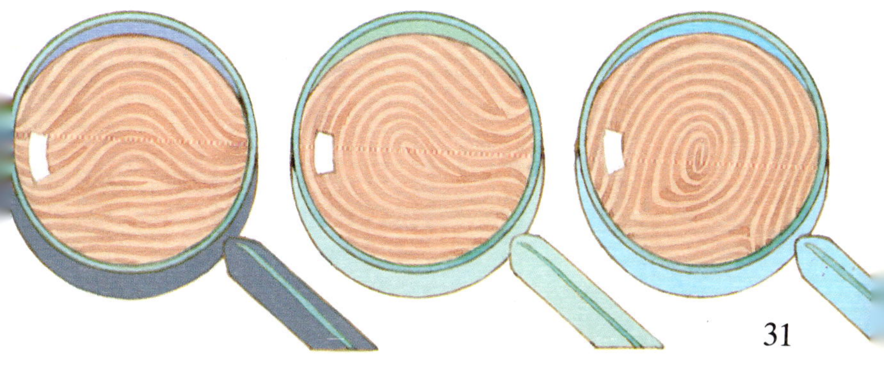

Hair and nails

We have hair all over our bodies, except for our palms and the soles of our feet.

You see only part of the hair. The rest is under the skin. It is called the root. When you are cold, a little muscle pulls the hair upright. You have goose pimples!

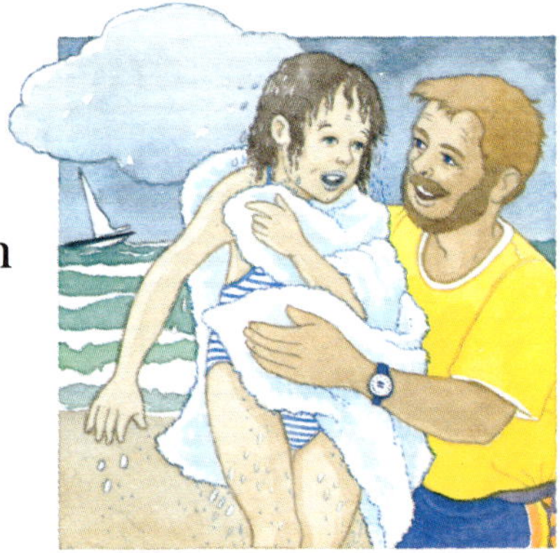

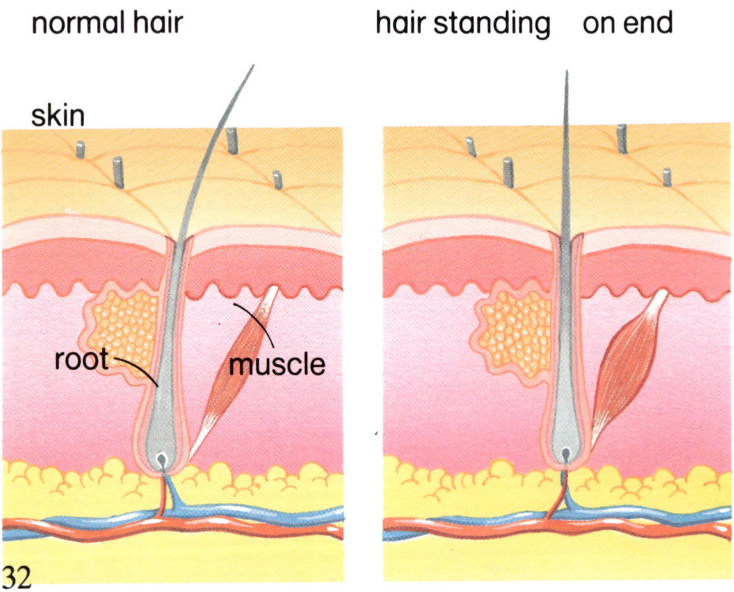

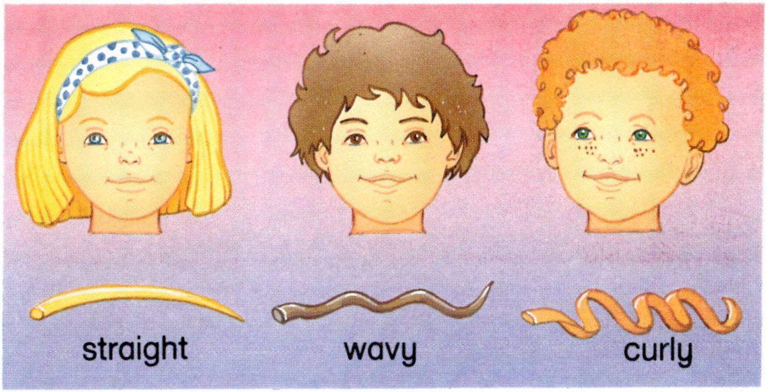

Hair grows out of tiny holes in our skin. Some people's hair grows straight, some wavy and some curly.

Hair is made of keratin. So are our nails. Nails protect our toes and fingertips.

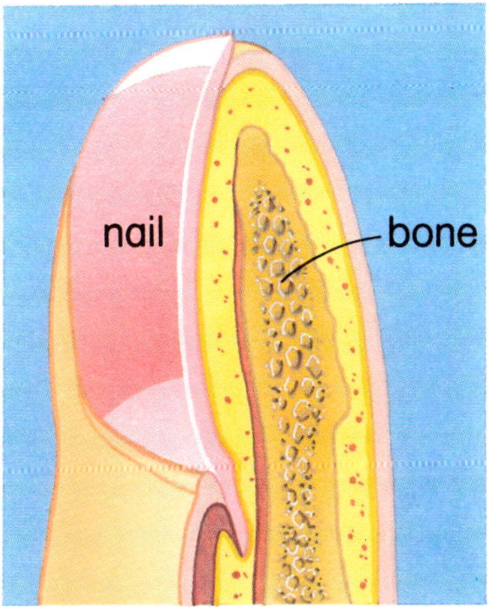

A cat's claws are its nails.

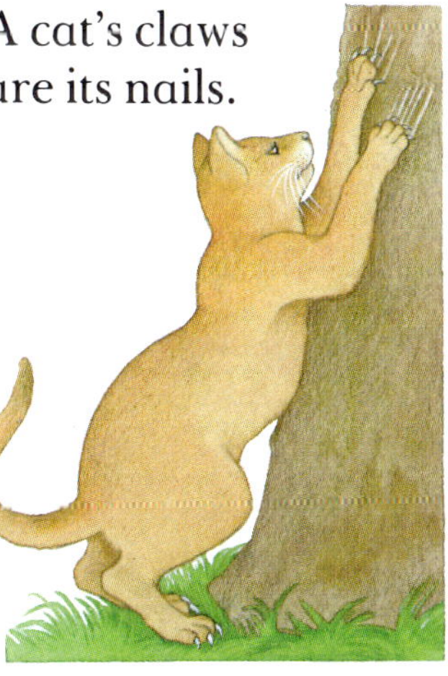

Muscles

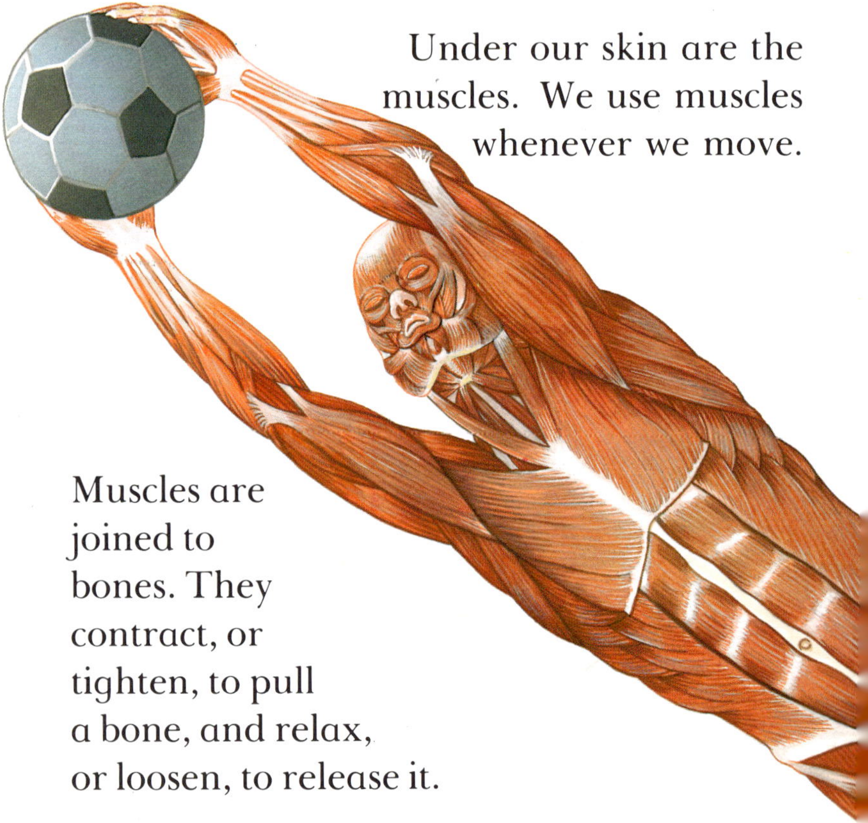

Under our skin are the muscles. We use muscles whenever we move.

Muscles are joined to bones. They contract, or tighten, to pull a bone, and relax, or loosen, to release it.

We have more than 650 muscles in our bodies. They move every part of the body, not just bones. The muscles in our face help us to smile, frown, wink and chew. The muscles in our chest help us to breathe.

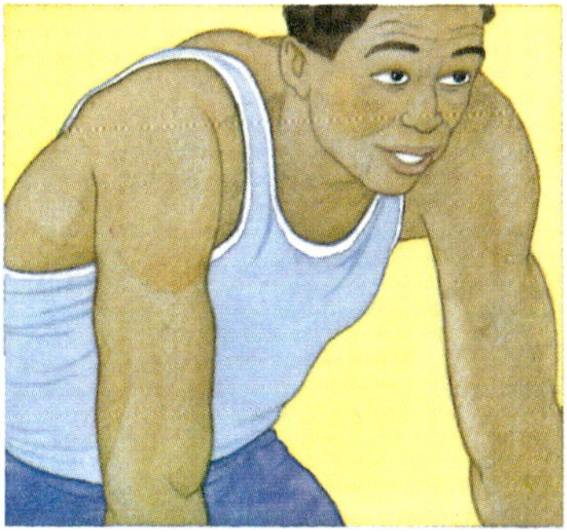

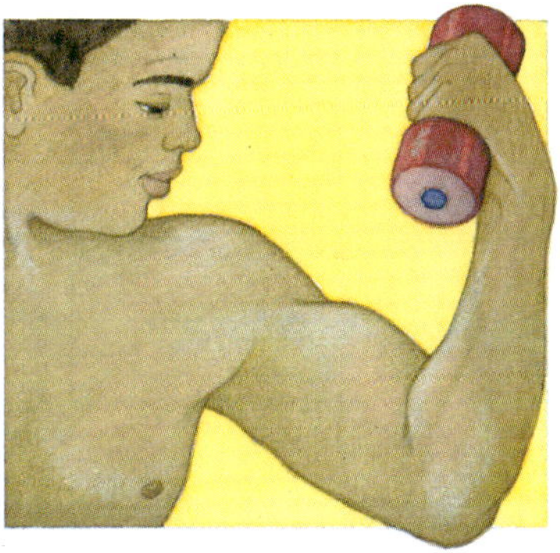

Muscles grow bigger and stronger with exercise and training.

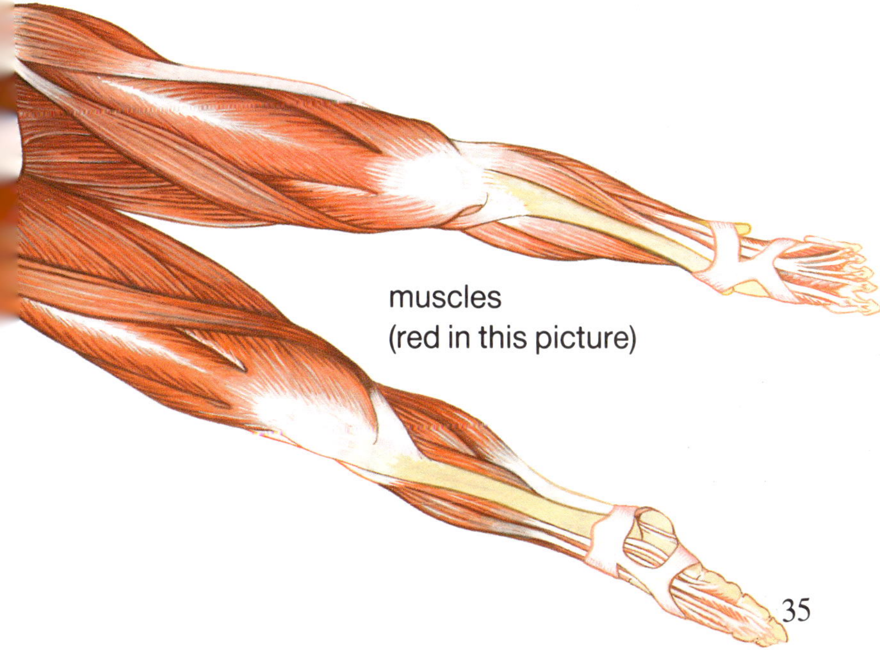

The skeleton

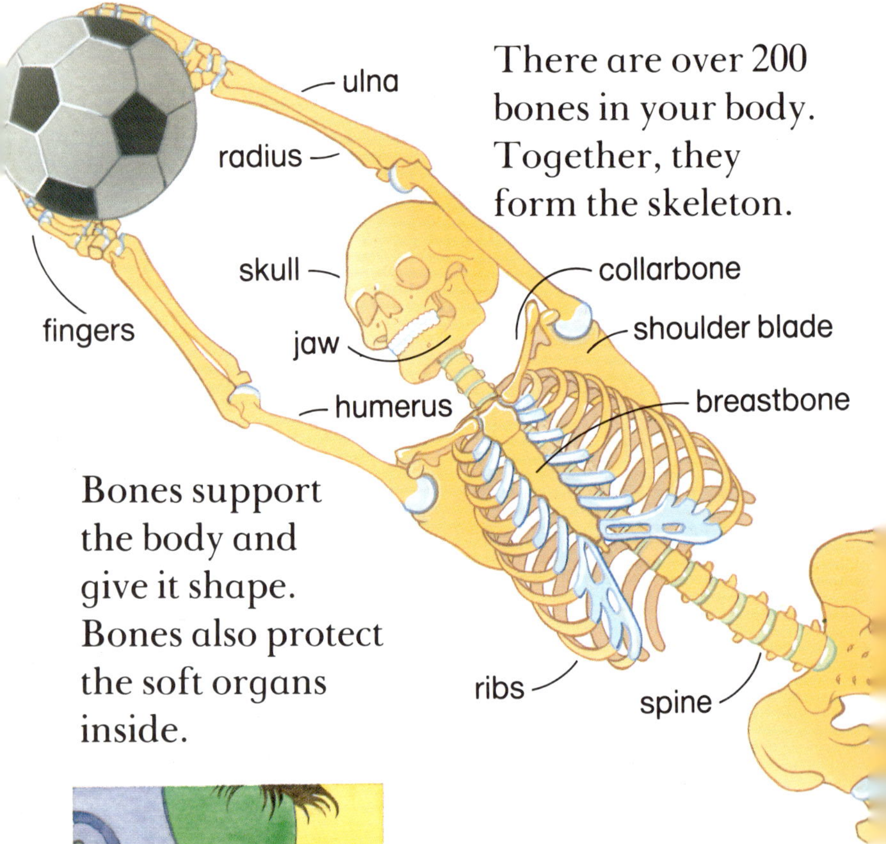

There are over 200 bones in your body. Together, they form the skeleton.

Bones support the body and give it shape. Bones also protect the soft organs inside.

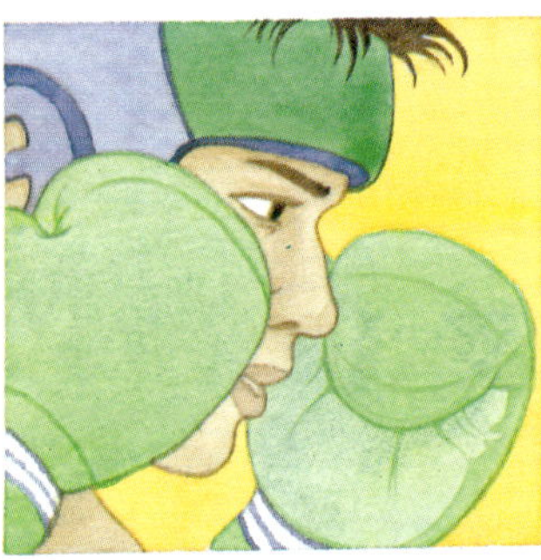

Your nose feels hard, but it is not all bone. The tip of it is a delicate piece of cartilage or gristle.

As you grow up, your bones grow longer and thicker. So you grow taller and heavier too.

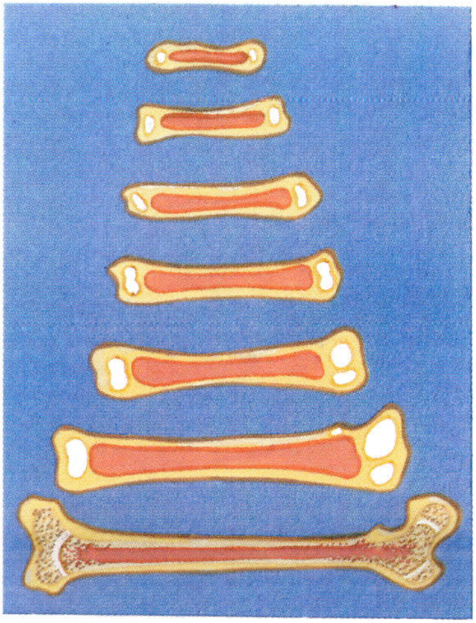

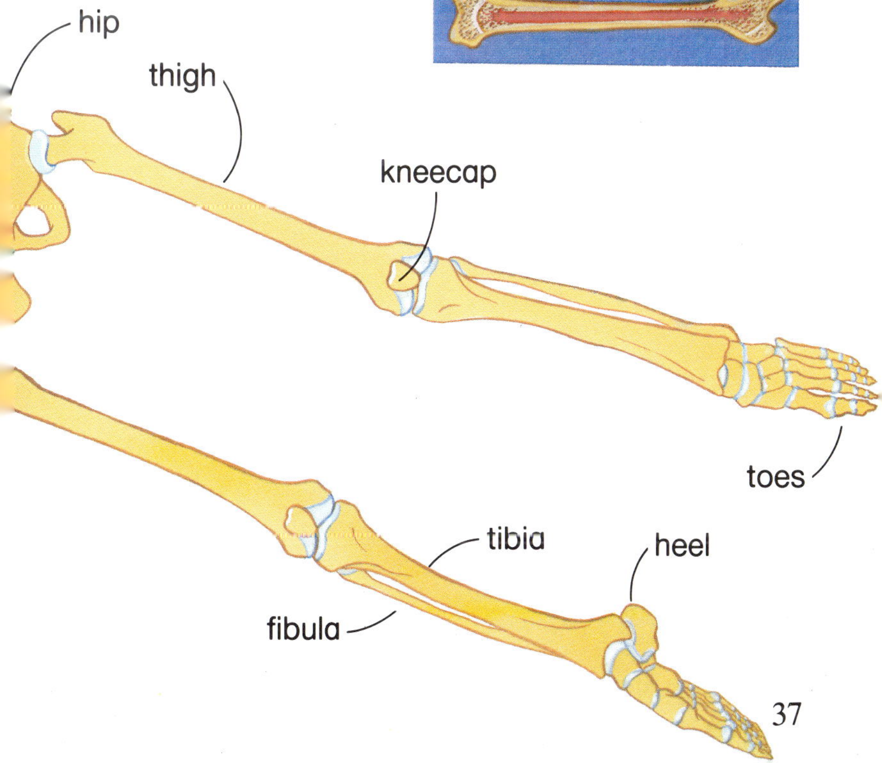

Bones and joints

Some bones fit together, others slide over each other. Our knees, spine, shoulders and elbows are some of the joints where bones meet.

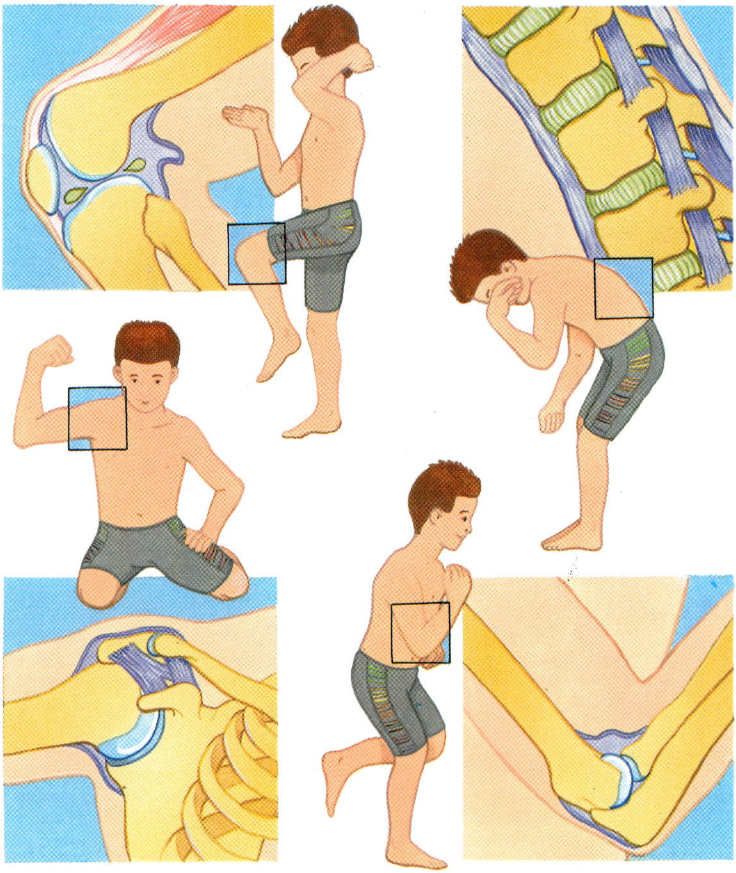

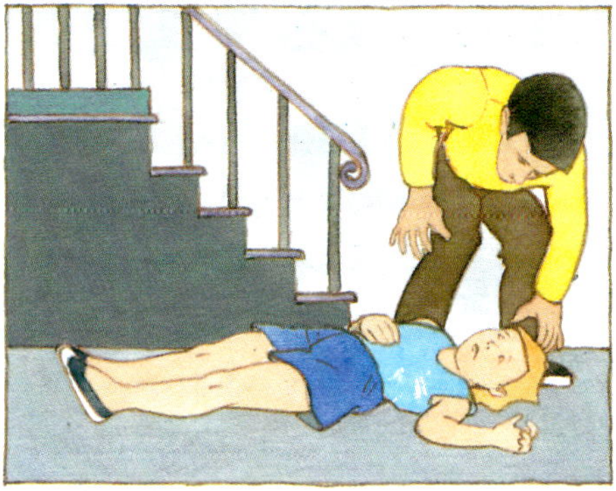

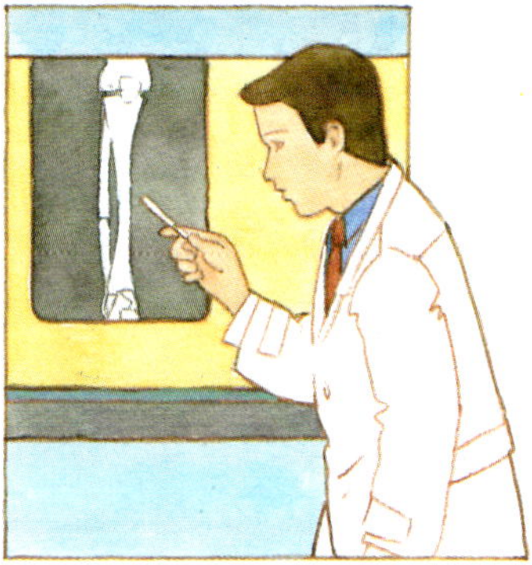

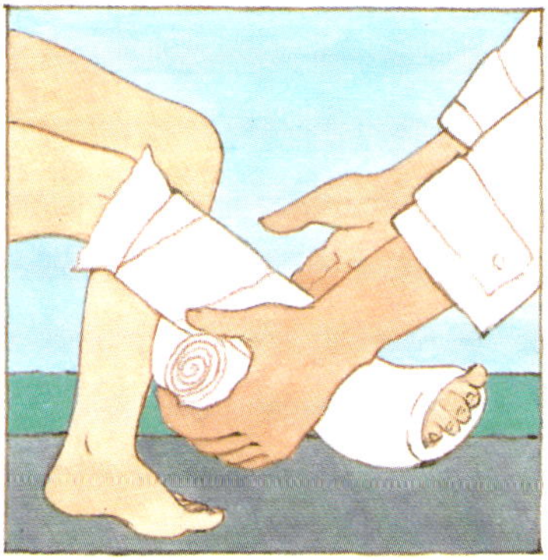

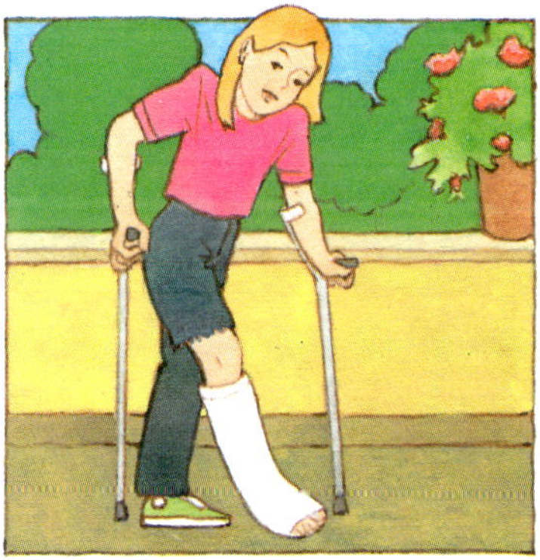

Although bones are strong, they may break in a fall. The doctor looks at the fracture, or break, on an X-ray photograph.

Then the injured part of the body may be wrapped in plaster, to hold the bone straight while it grows back together again.

The brain

The brain inside your head is the most important part of your body.

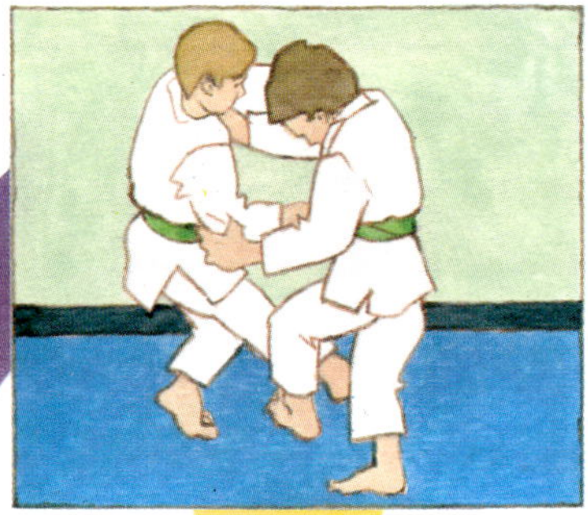

Your brain tells your body how to work. (Pages 100–101 show you how.)

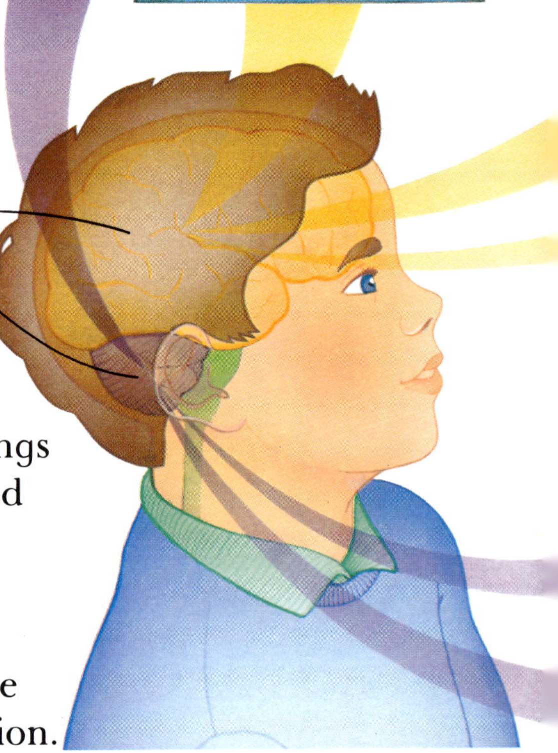

Your brain helps your body to feel things and to think and learn. Part of your brain, the cerebellum, controls balance and co-ordination.

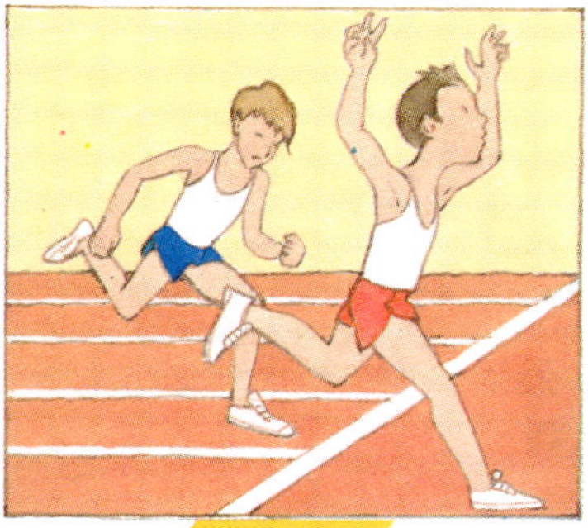

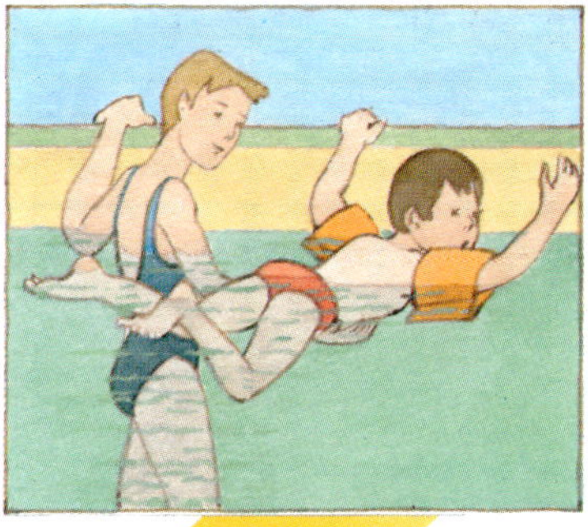

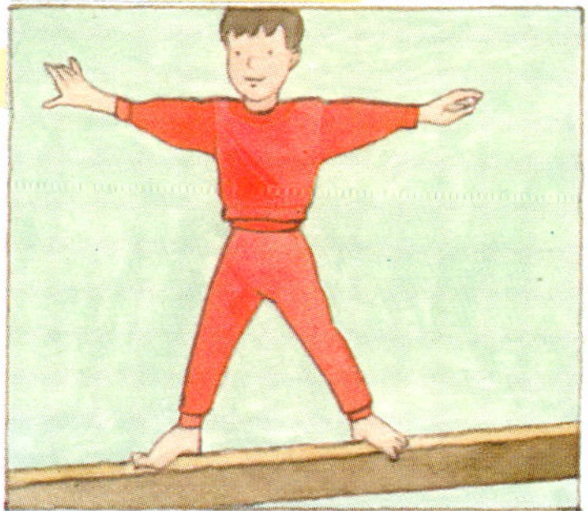

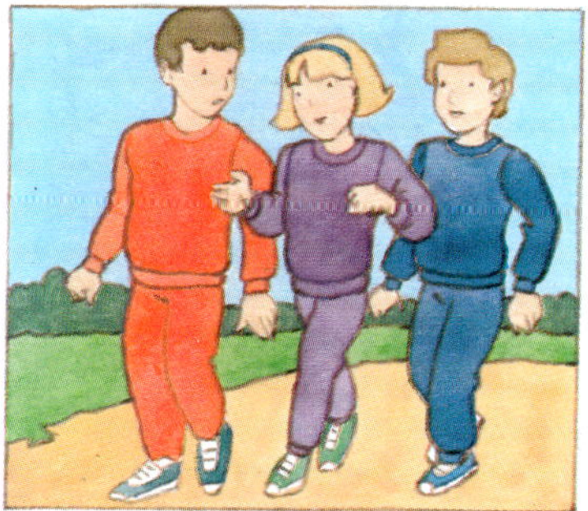

Other organs

The brain is one of the soft organs inside your body. The other organs all have special tasks of their own. They help the body to work properly.

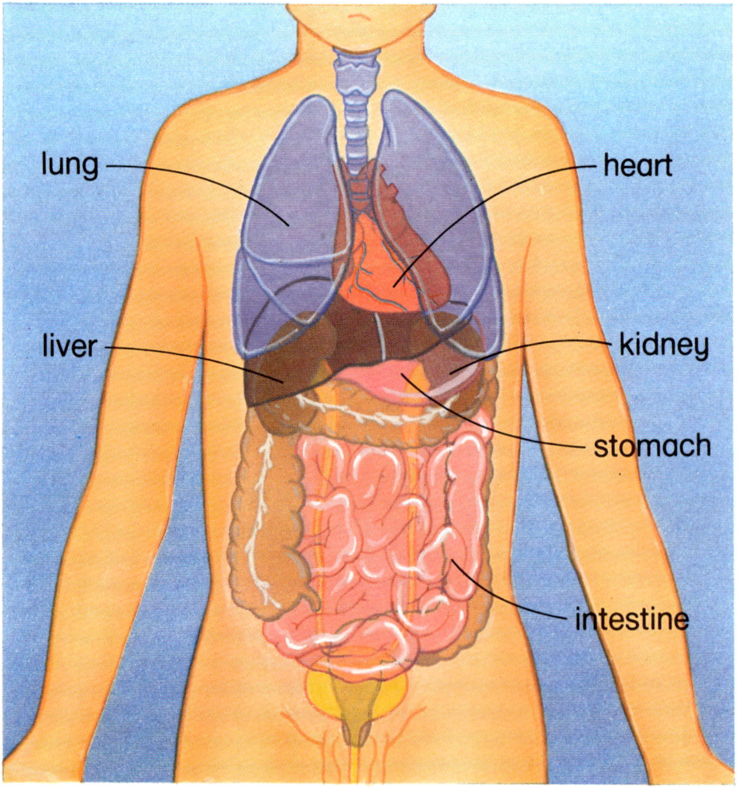

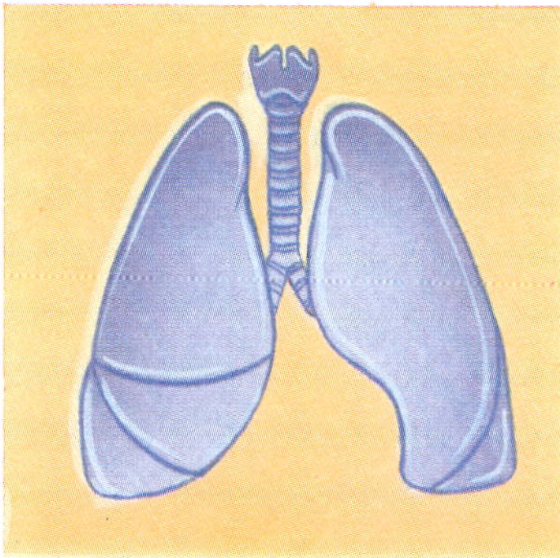

The lungs supply blood with oxygen.

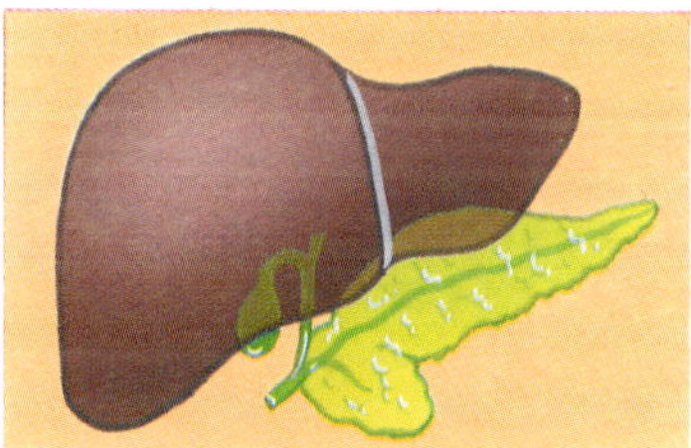

The liver helps us to digest our food.

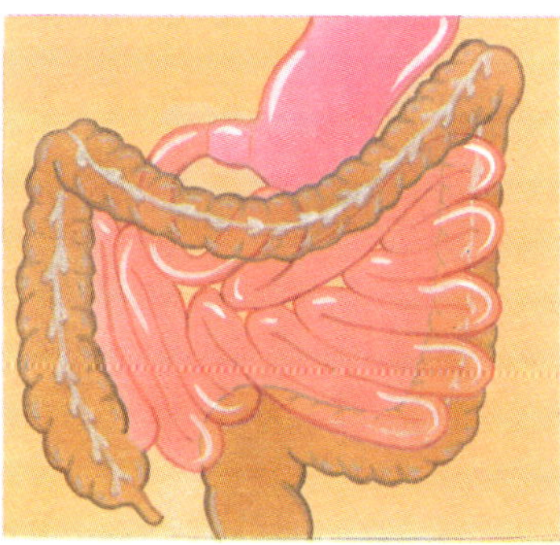

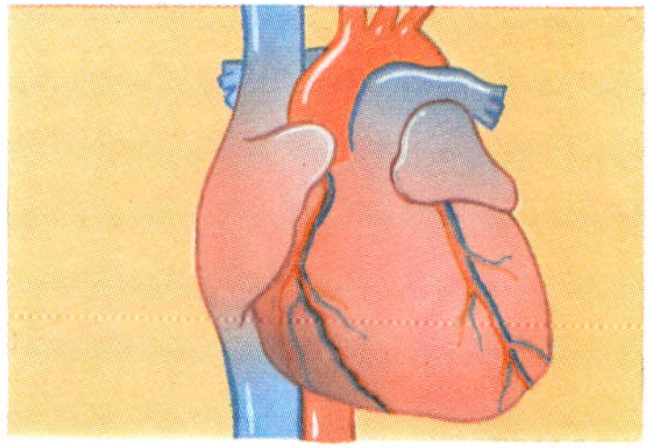

The heart pumps blood around the body.

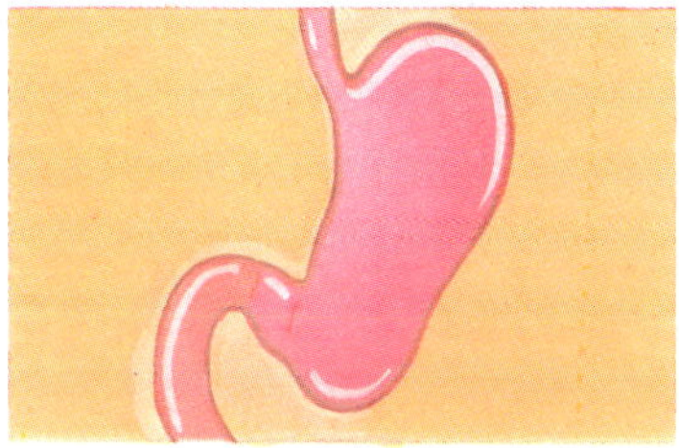

The stomach mashes food into a pulp.

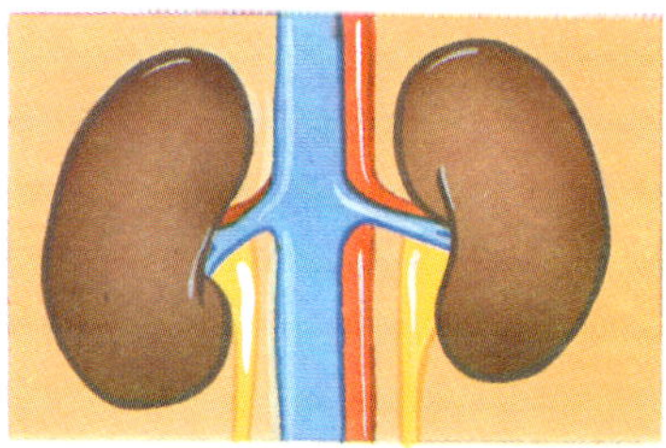

◀ The intestines pass food into the blood.

▲ Two kidneys help to get rid of waste.

Amazing facts

More than 200 muscles go into action when you take a step, but only 15 when you smile!

We have 300 bones at birth, but only 208 when we are adults. This is because some bones join together as we grow up.

Fingernails grow twice as fast as toenails, about one millimetre a week. Human nails and hair are made of keratin. So are reptiles' scales and birds' feathers.

We lose about fifty hairs every day.

Life story

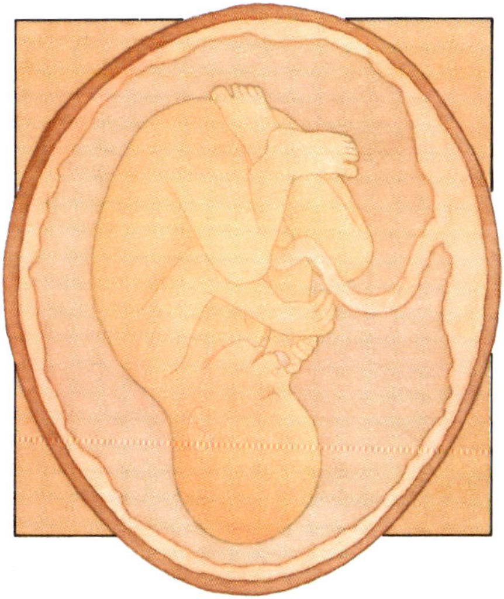

Where do you come from?

The body is made of millions of tiny living parts called cells – bone cells and skin cells, brain cells and blood cells, cells for every part of your body.

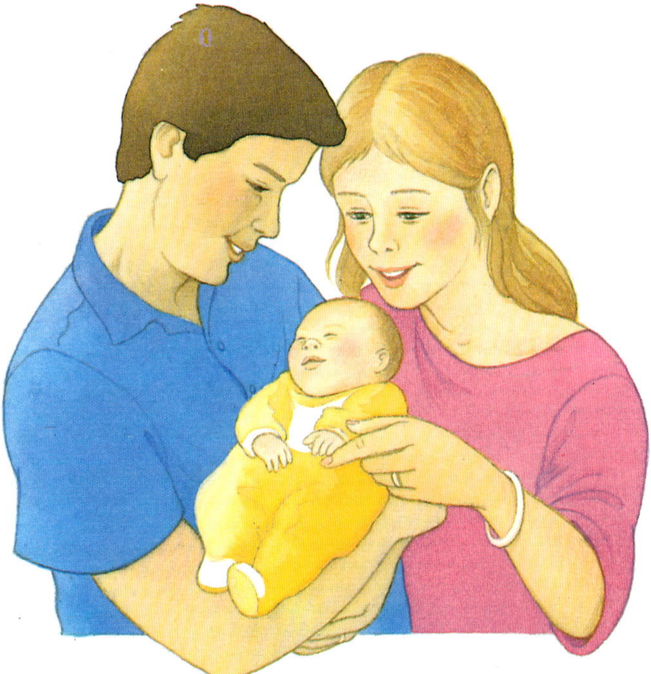

But we all began as just one cell inside our mother's body, before we were born. Every baby is made by a man and a woman. They are the baby's parents.

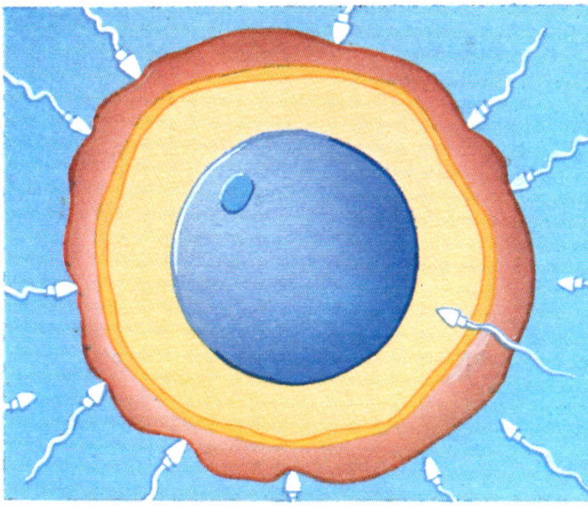

A sperm from the father enters an egg inside the mother.

Now the egg is fertilized. It is the first cell of the baby.

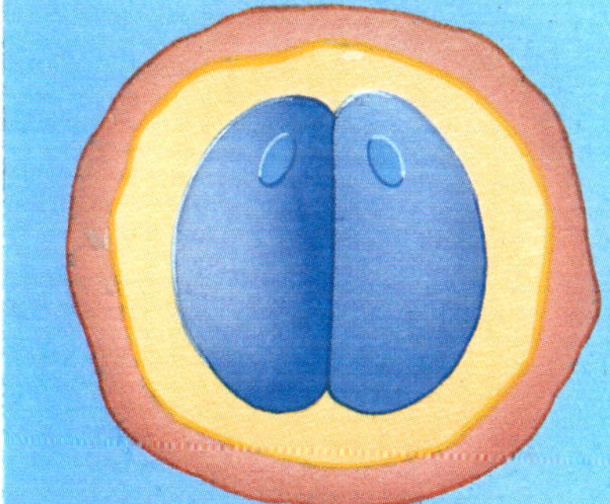

The egg is even smaller than a dot made by a pencil.

The egg splits into two cells, and then into four, and so on.

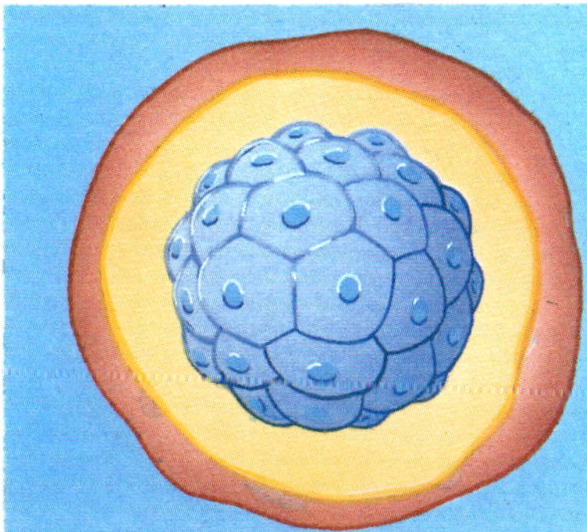

So the egg grows bigger and bigger.

The egg moves to a part of the mother called the womb. This is the start of her pregnancy.

Boy or girl?

What will the baby look like? The answer is in the genes.

Genes are special instructions in each cell which tell it what to do. Everyone has two sets of genes, one from the father's sperm and one from the mother's egg. The colour of the baby's hair and eyes, how tall it will grow, whether it is a boy or a girl – everything is decided by the genes.

A doctor or a midwife checks that the pregnancy is going well. A scanning machine shows the baby inside the womb. If they want to, the parents can find out if the baby is a boy or a girl.

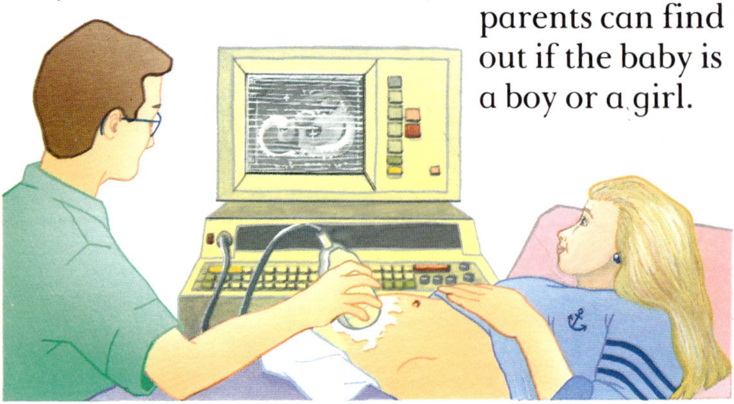

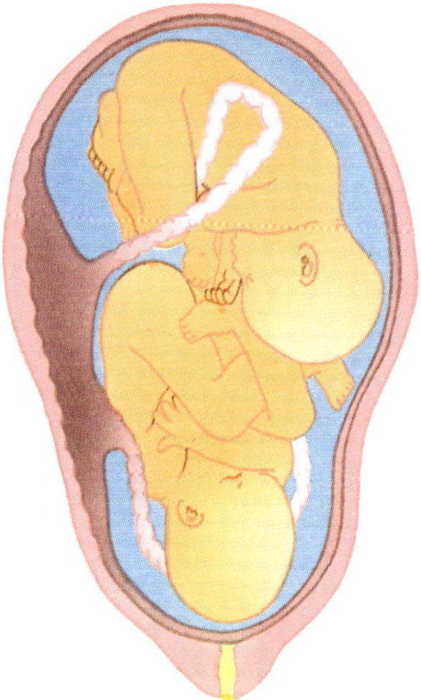

Sometimes a mother has
two babies from one egg.
These are identical twins,
two boys or two girls
who will look just like
each other.

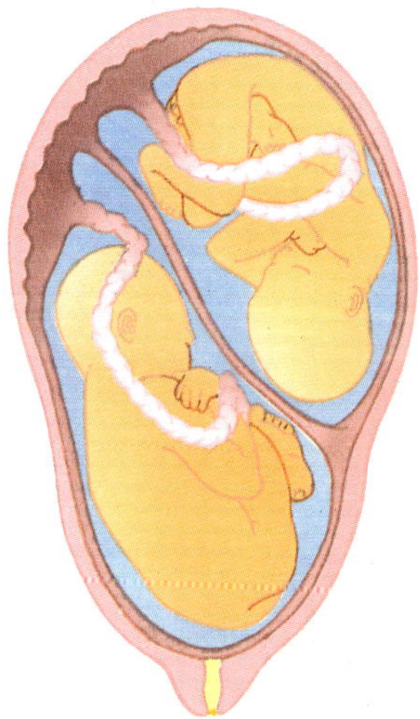

Or she may have twins
from two eggs. These
twins are not identical.

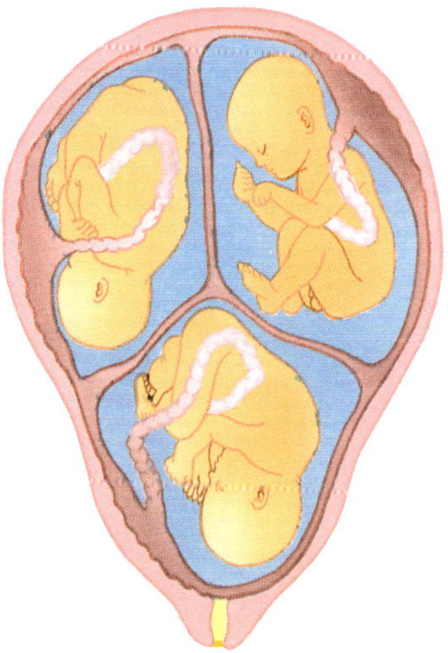

It is very rare, but
there may even be
three, four, five or six
babies!

Nine months for a baby

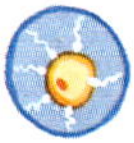

The baby grows in a bag of warm liquid in the mother's womb. It gets all the food and oxygen it needs from its mother's body, through a tube called the umbilical cord.

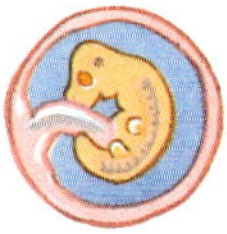

At one month, the baby's heart is beating. The baby is no bigger than a pea.

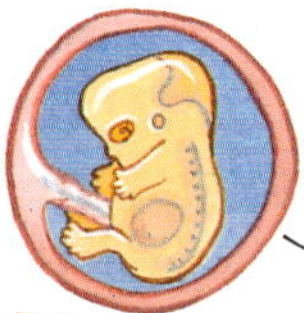

At three months, it is about six centimetres long and looks more like a baby.

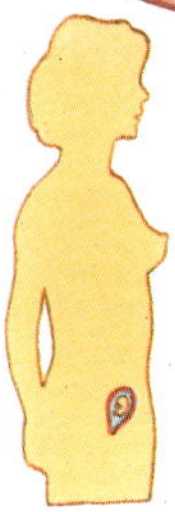

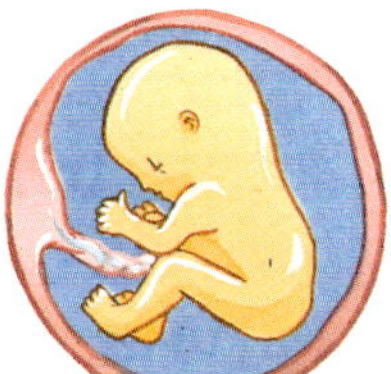

At four months, it can move about.

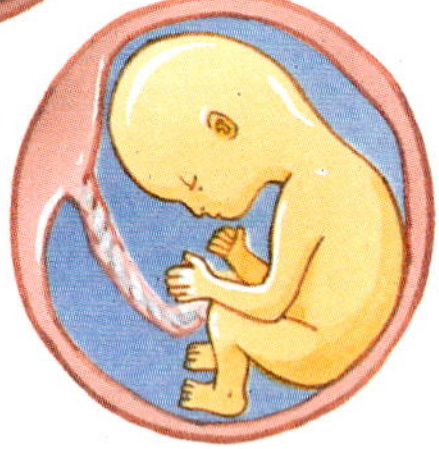

At five months, it sucks its thumb.

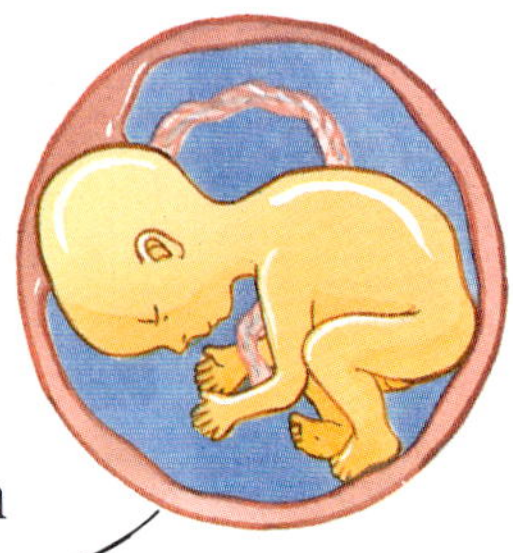

At six months, it can hear sounds.

At nine months, the baby is ready to come out of its mother's womb.

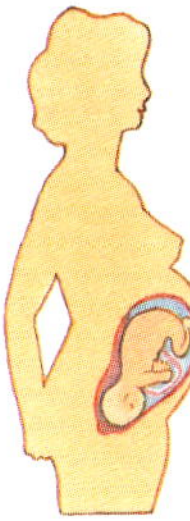

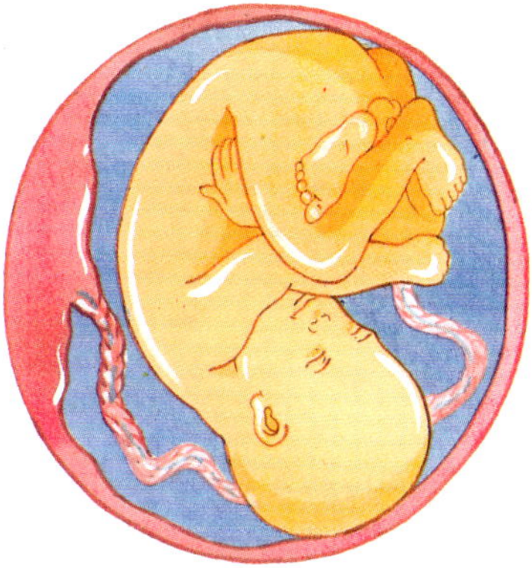

Then it usually turns upside down.

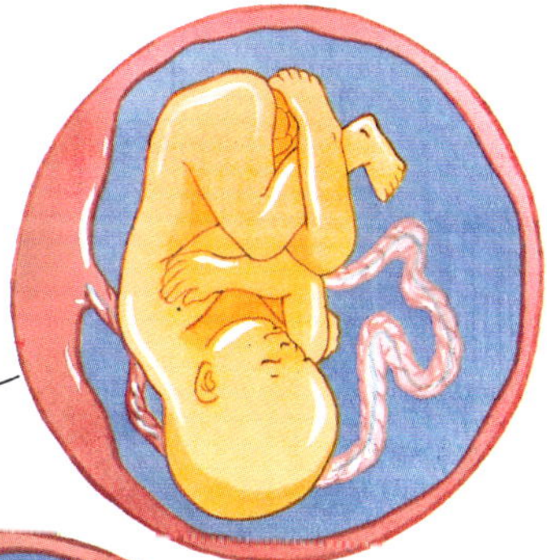

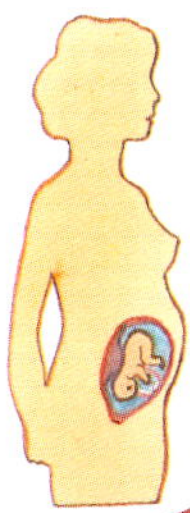

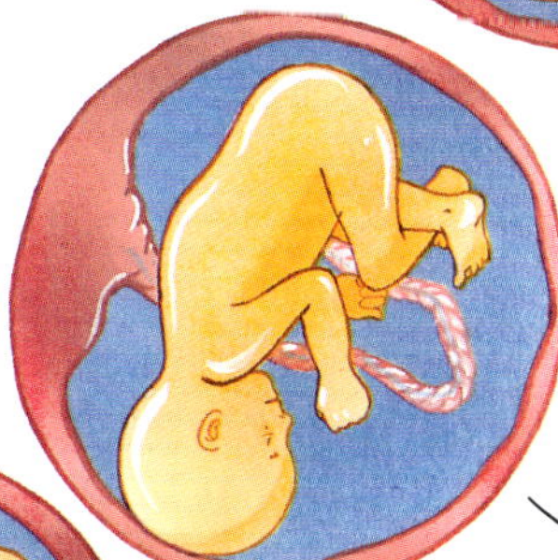

At eight months, it can taste things.

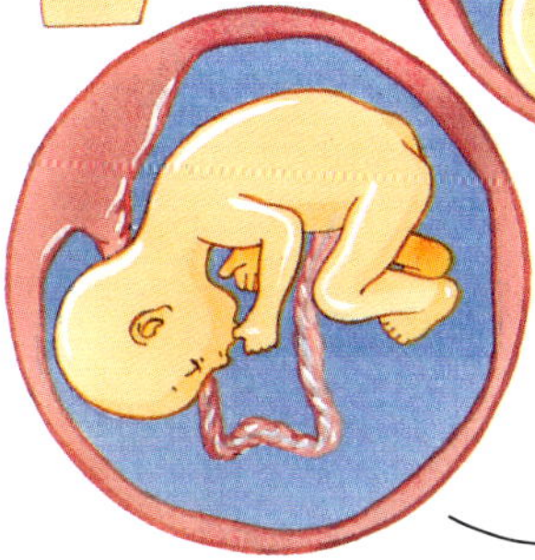

At seven months, it opens its eyes. It can kick strongly.

The birth

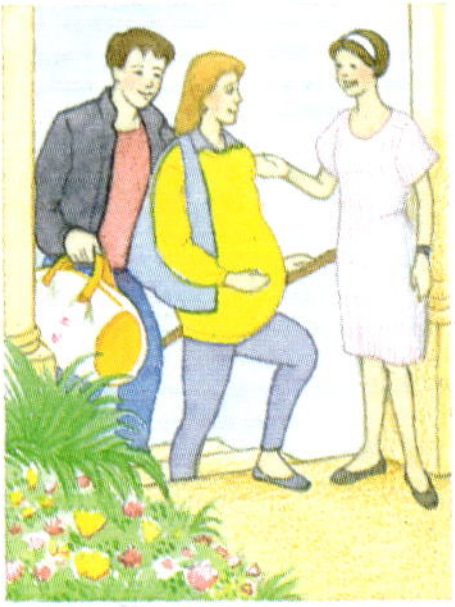

When the baby is ready to be born, the mother can go to hospital to give birth.
Her muscles help to push the baby out. Usually the baby comes out head first.

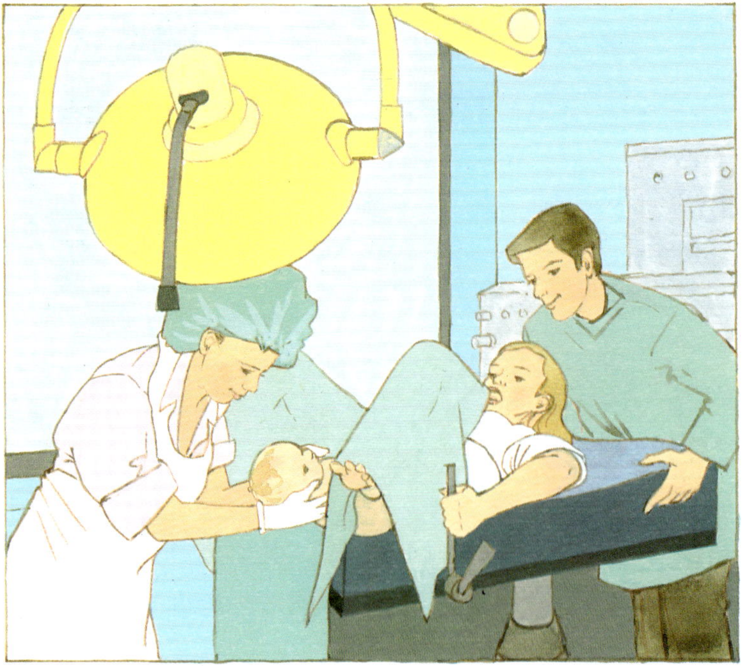

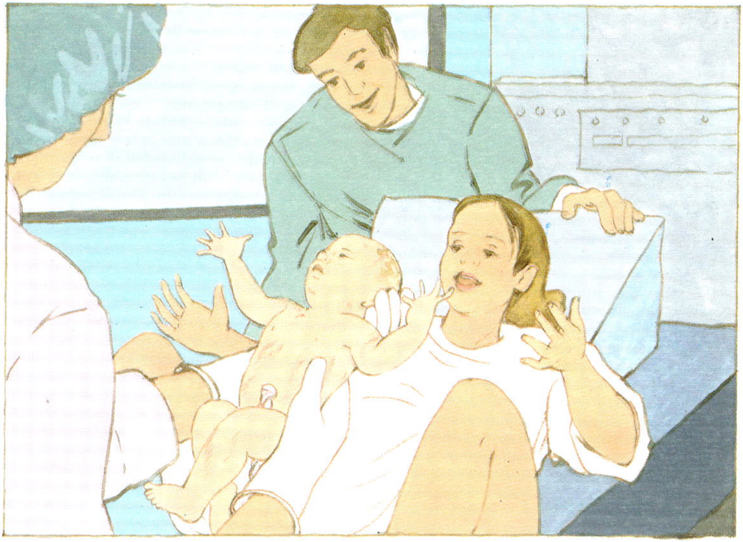

The doctor or the midwife helps the baby to come out. The baby takes its first breath and cries. It does not need the umbilical cord after it is born. So the cord is cut off.

The umbilical cord's scar becomes our navel, or 'tummy button'.

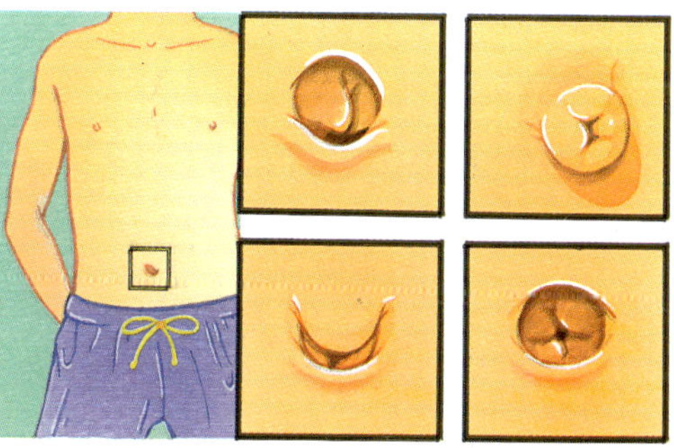

Baby days

A brand-new baby needs a lot of care and love.

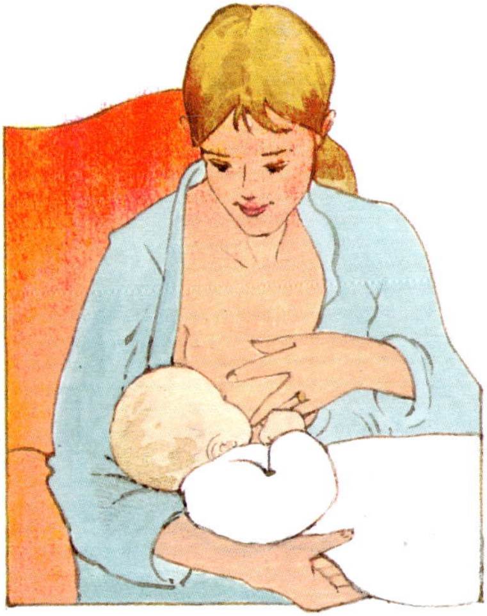

At first, it sleeps a lot. When it is hungry, it cries for its mother's milk or its bottle.

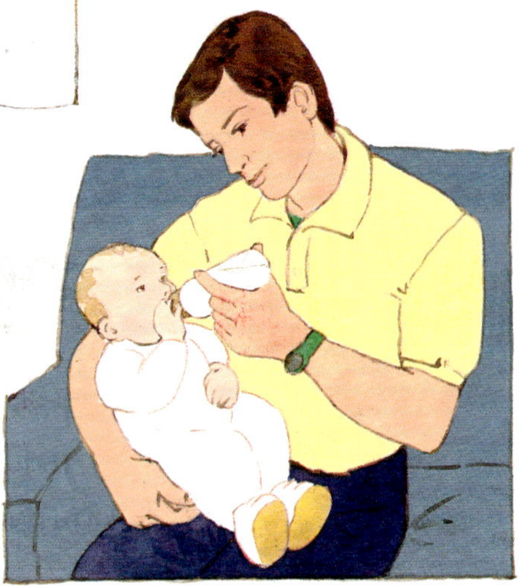

The baby likes being held by its parents.
It recognizes their voices and their smell.

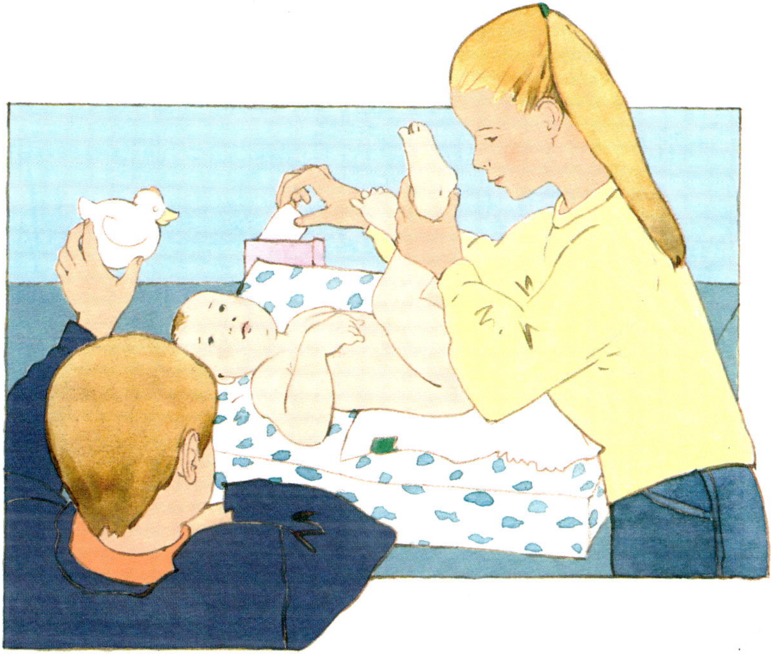

The baby looks at things nearby. It enjoys its bath and clean nappies, and it smiles.

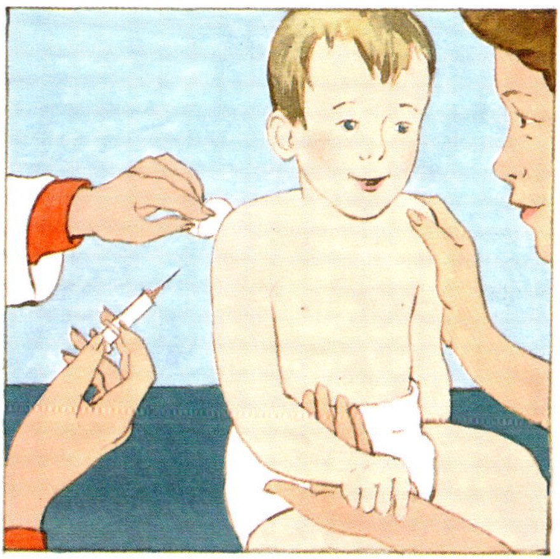

Vaccinations protect the baby from diseases.

Childhood

The baby grows. It does more and more things by itself.

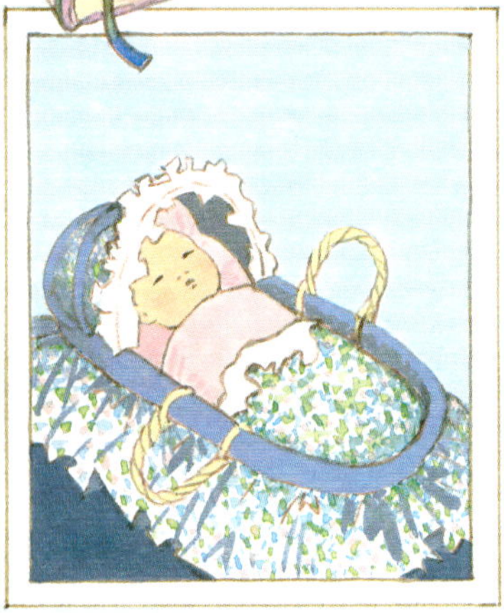

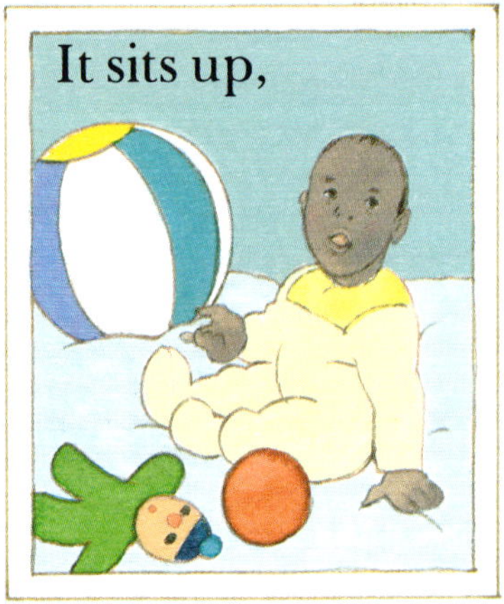

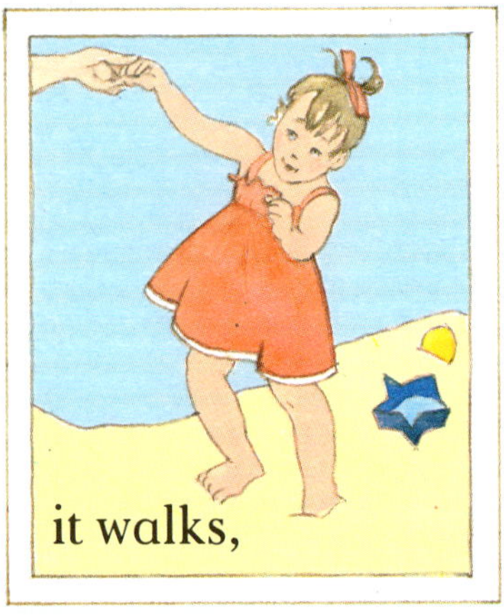

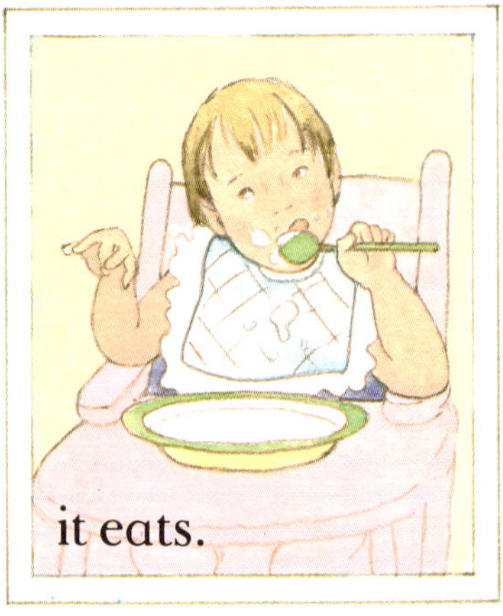

The baby grows into a child. Children are learning things all the time: riding their first bike, going to school, playing games and meeting other people.

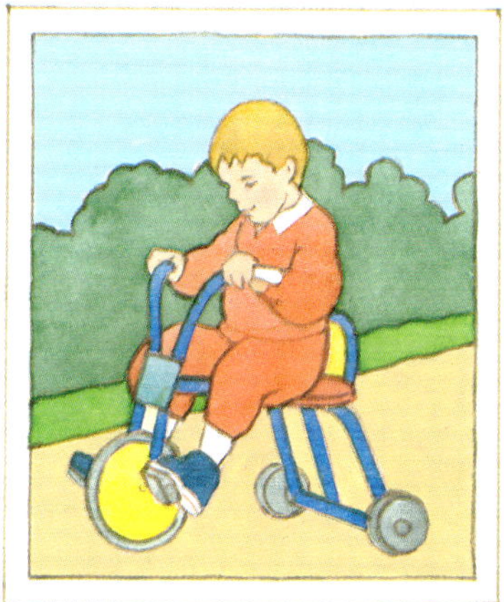

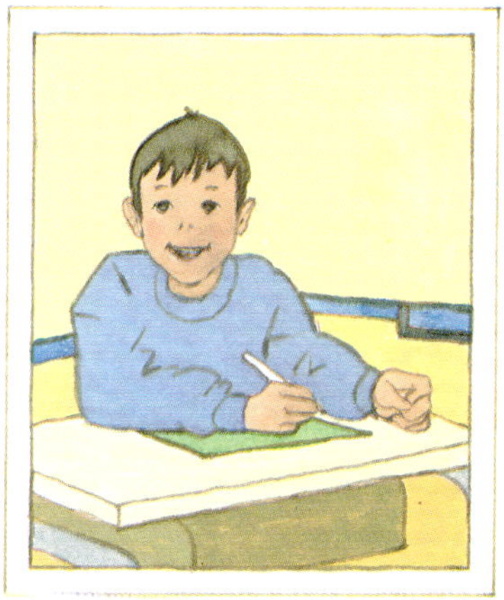

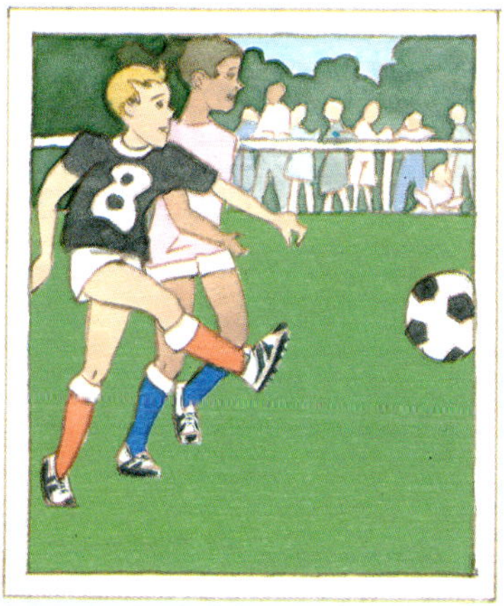

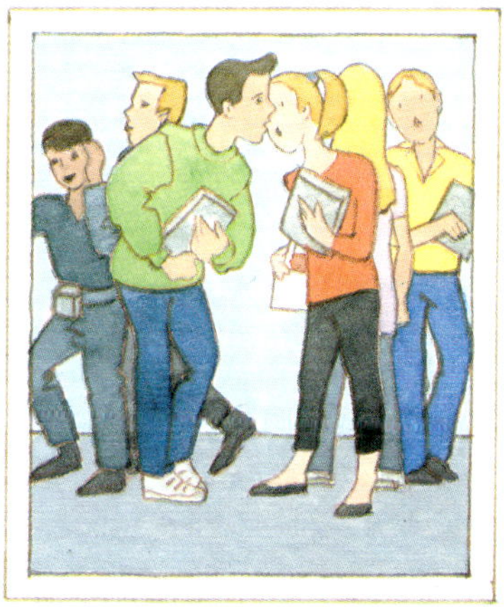

Growing up

Children grow into teenagers and adults. By the time they are about eighteen years old, their bodies have stopped growing.

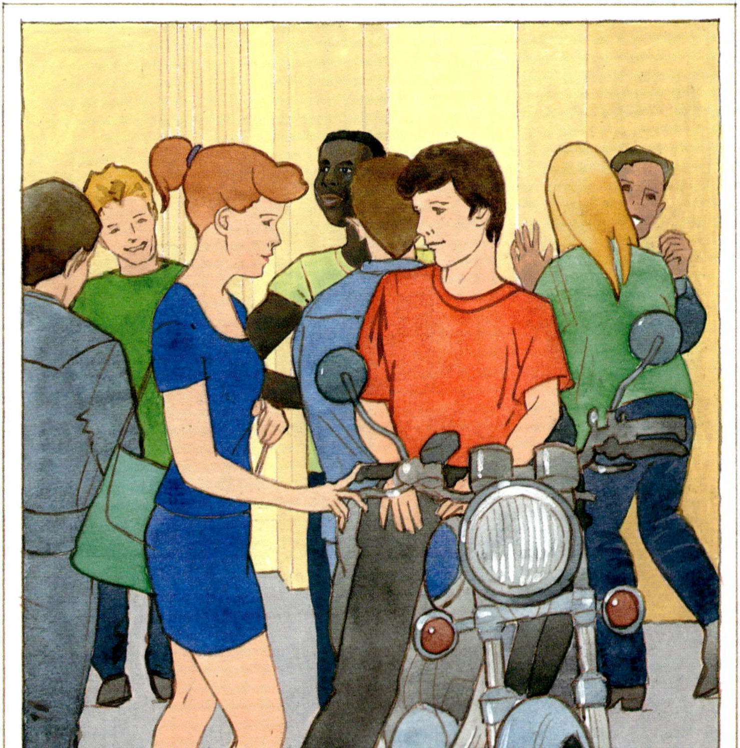

People start work, and they fall in love.

If they want to, a man and woman can live together and start a family.

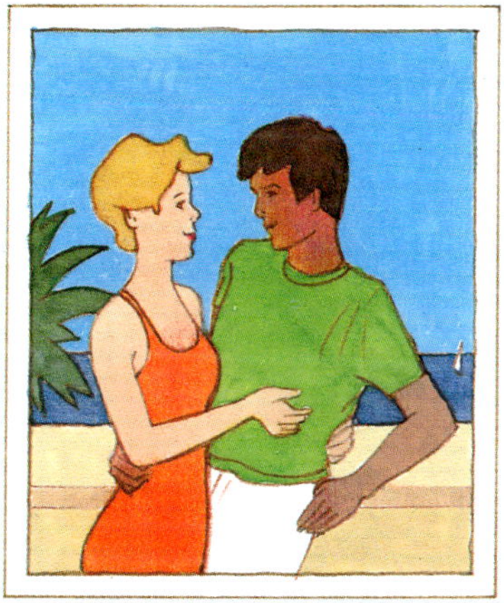
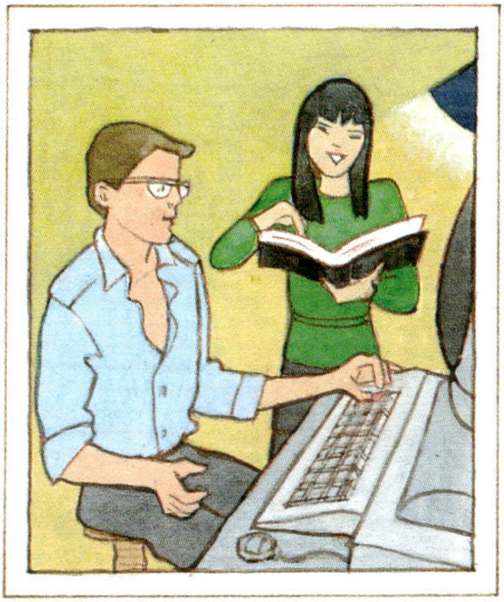
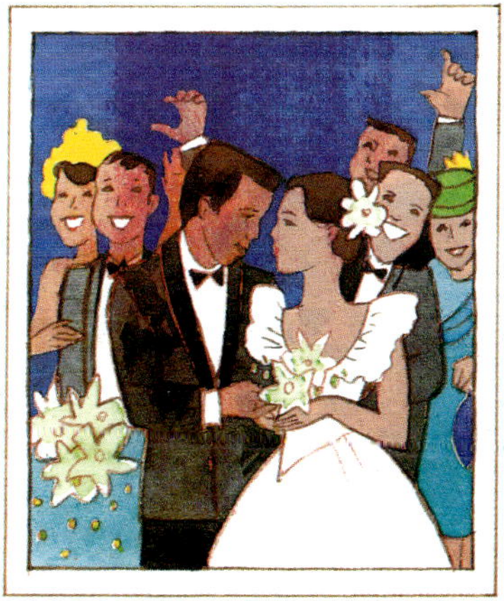
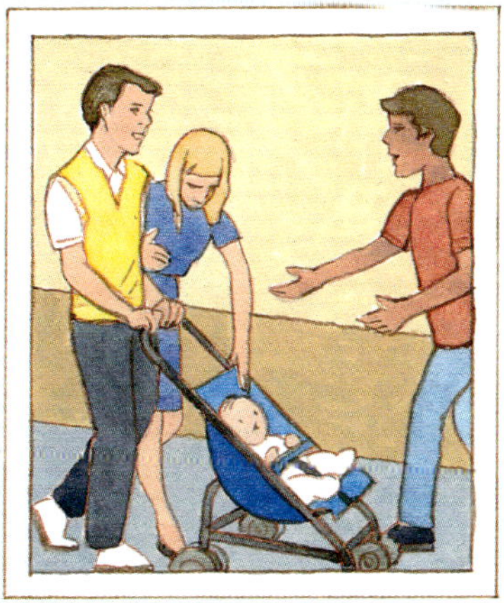

Growing old

People have busy lives, working, studying and bringing up a family.

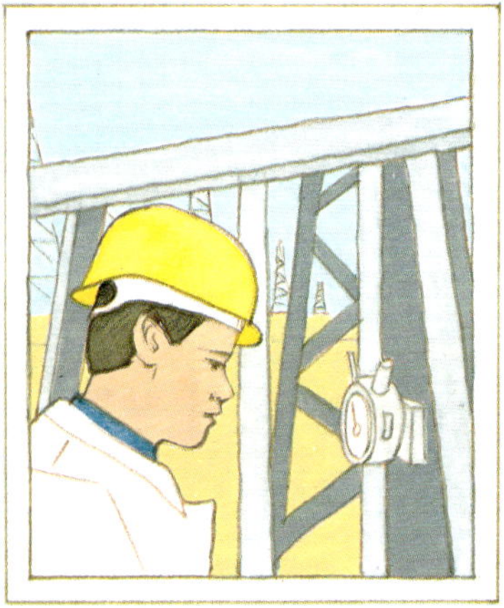

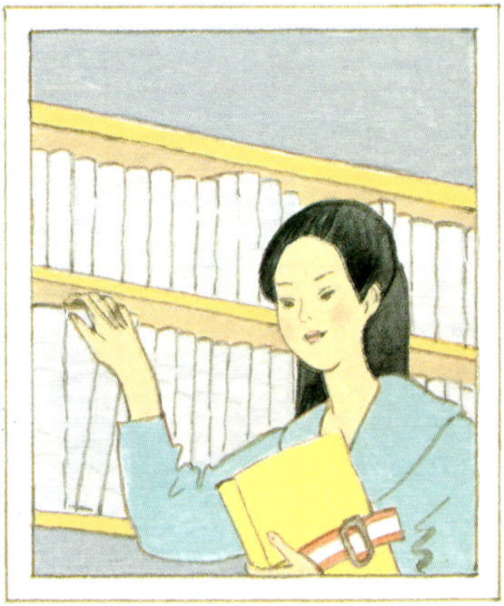

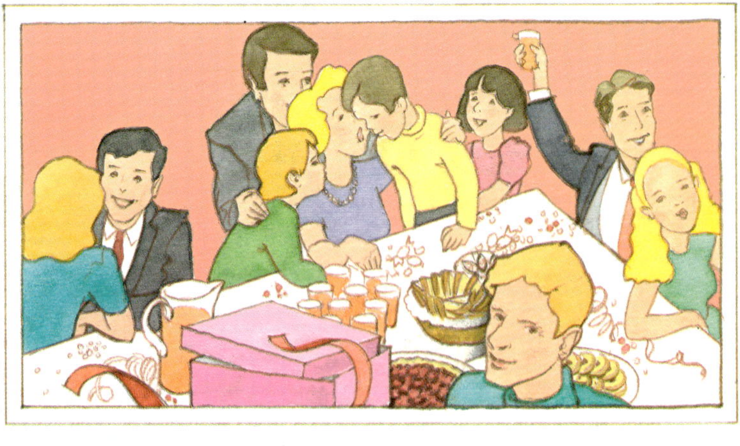

As the body grows older, the muscles get weaker, so they get tired more easily.

When people die, those who loved them can remember them long after they have gone.

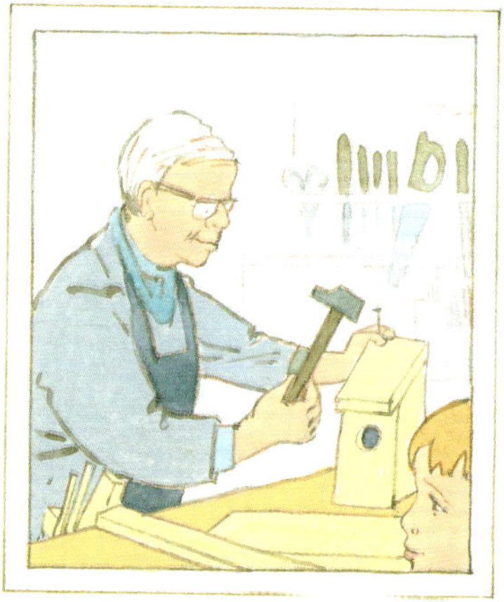

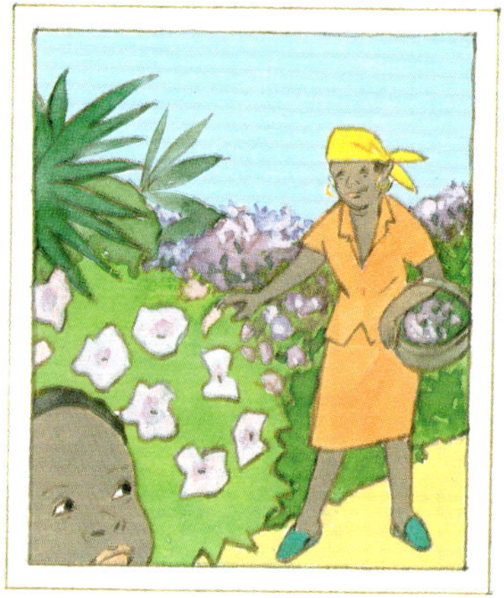

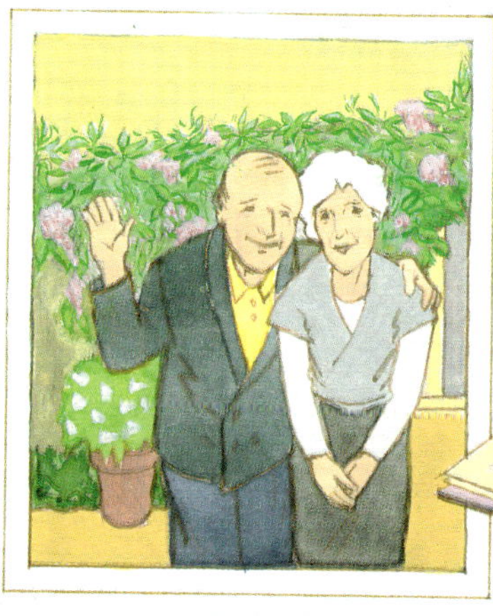

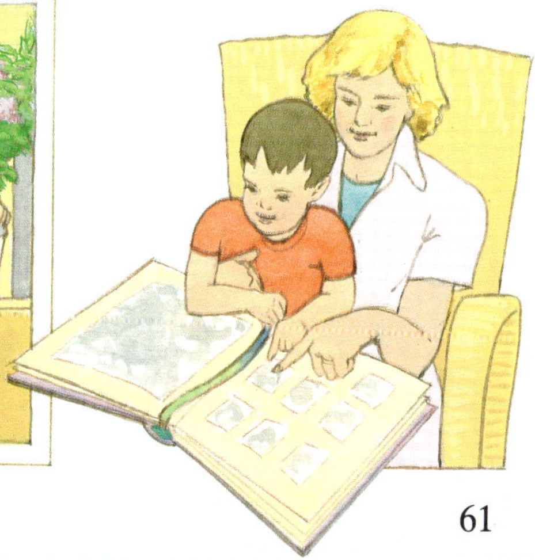

Amazing facts

An adult body has about 50 billion cells – remember, all those cells begin with just one cell, the fertilized egg.

The egg is the biggest cell in the body. But it is only one fifth of a millimetre wide.

Which lives longest: a dog, a human or an elephant? A human! The oldest person ever lived to be 121.

Around the world, 140 babies are born every minute.

The senses

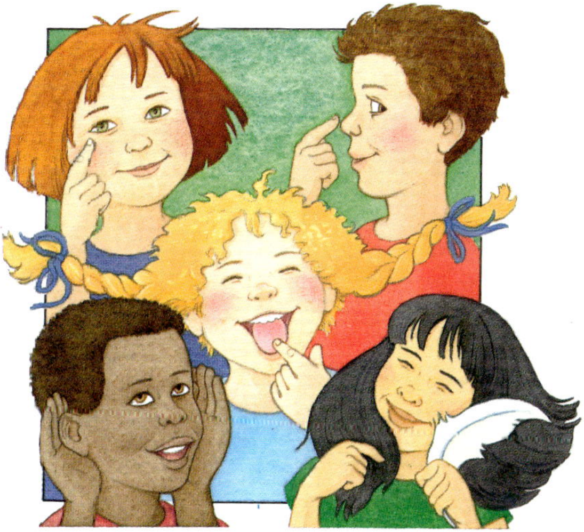

Hearing

We hear sounds all the time. They are invisible waves in the air. Some sounds are pleasant, some are not. But they all give us information about the world around us.

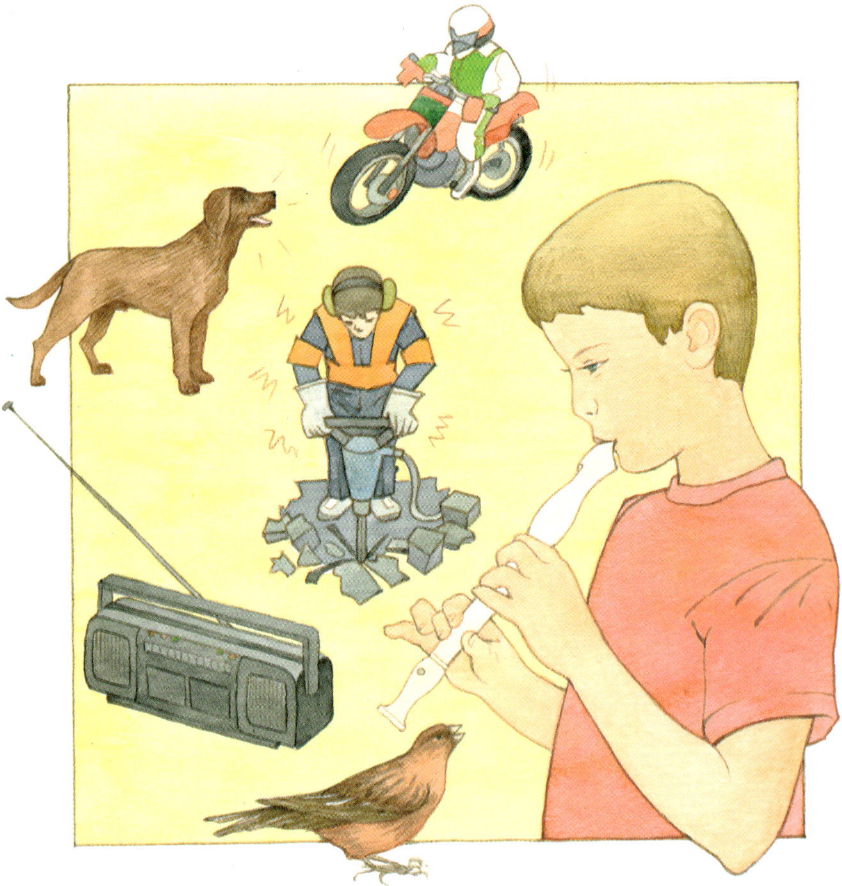

We can see only part of the ear. The rest is inside the head. Sounds enter the ear, and make the eardrum vibrate. This makes tiny bones move. Then a nerve carries the message to the brain.

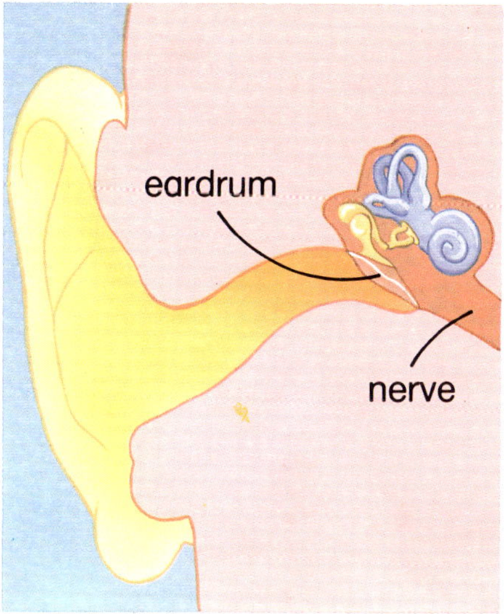

The brain tells us what we are hearing.

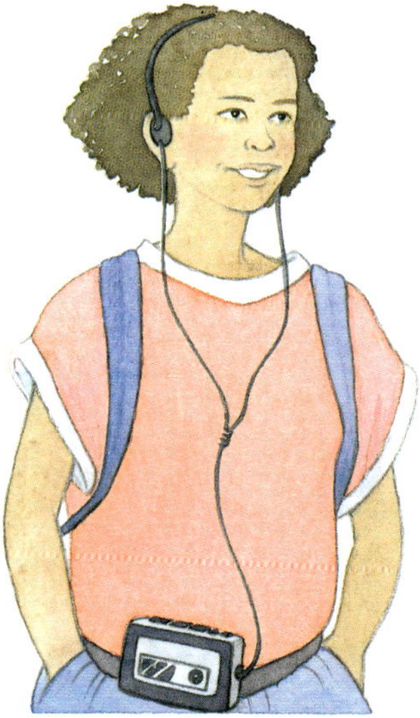

A hearing aid makes sounds louder, to help people who cannot hear well.

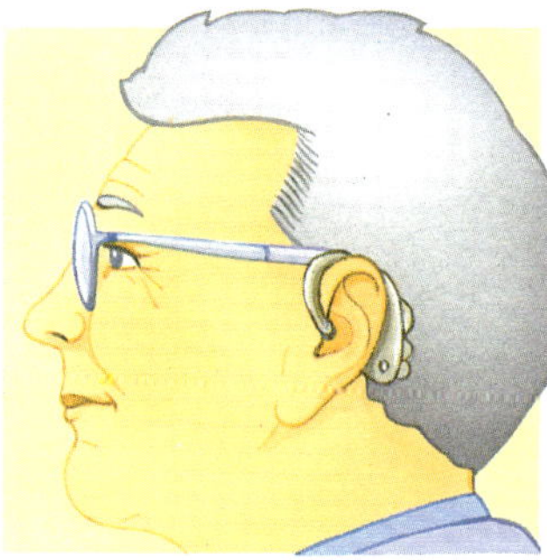

Smell

We use the nose for breathing, and for smelling. Smells float in the air. Although they are invisible, we can tell what they are. We like some smells, but not others!

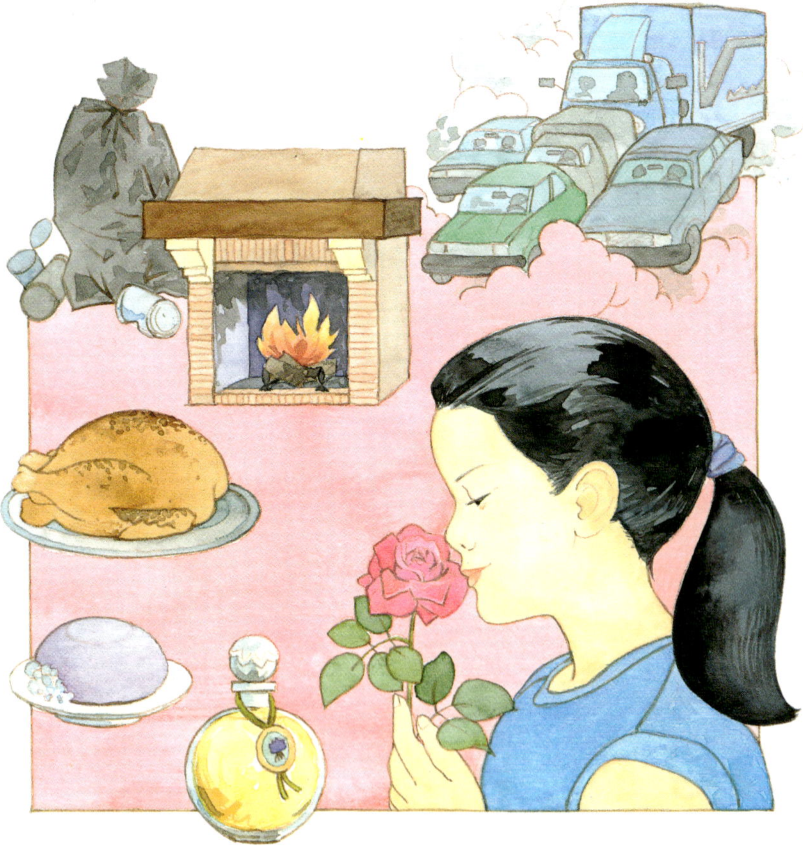

When a smell reaches the back of your nose, nerves carry the information to the brain. The brain decides what the smell is.

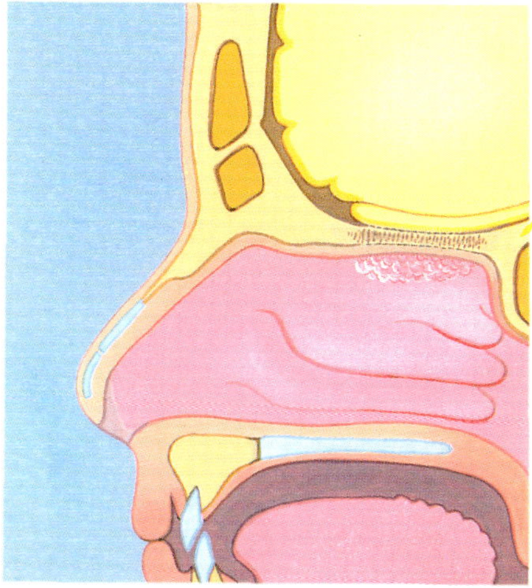

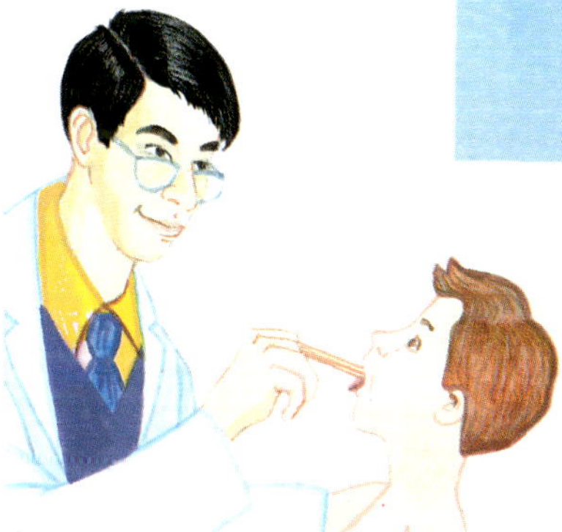

Some doctors look after only the ears, nose and throat.

Our sense of smell helps our sense of taste. That is why it is difficult to taste things when you have a cold and a blocked-up nose.

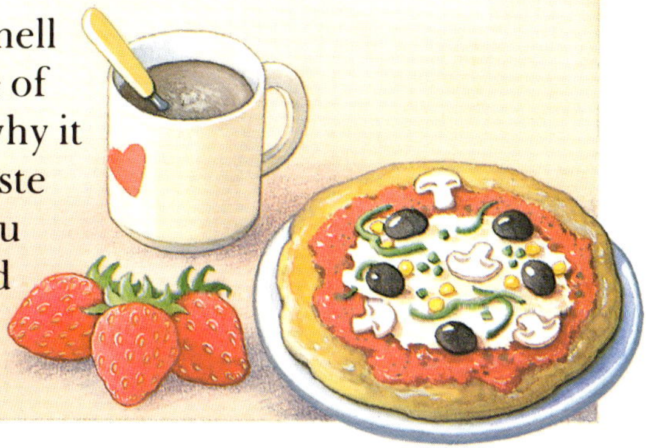

Touch

When we touch things, we can feel them. Our skin feels the heat of a cup of cocoa, the cold of ice, the prick of a thorn, the softness of a cat's fur.

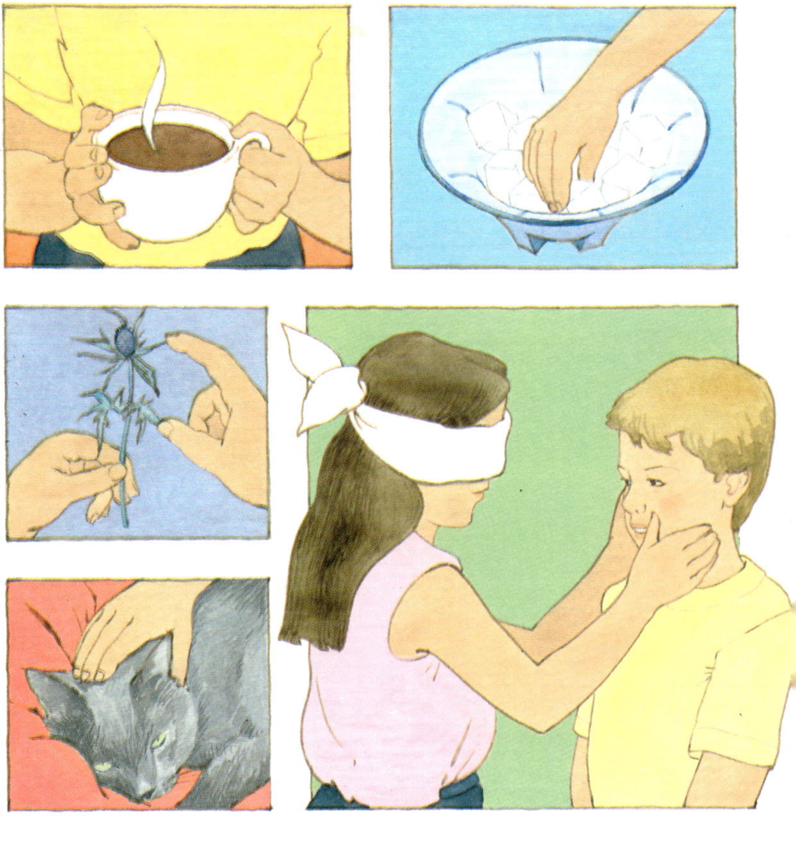

Tiny nerves in the skin send messages about things we touch to the brain.

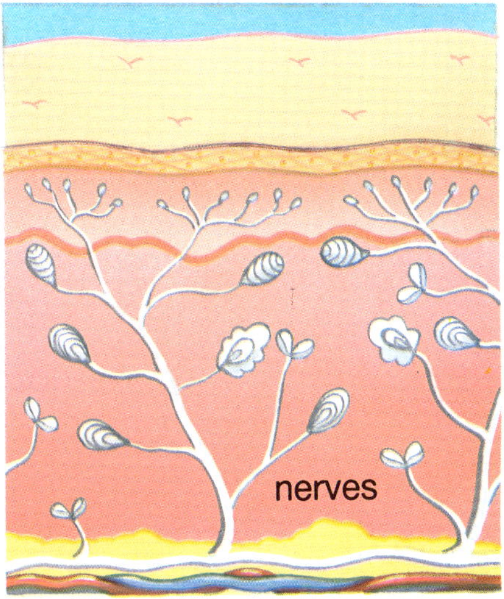

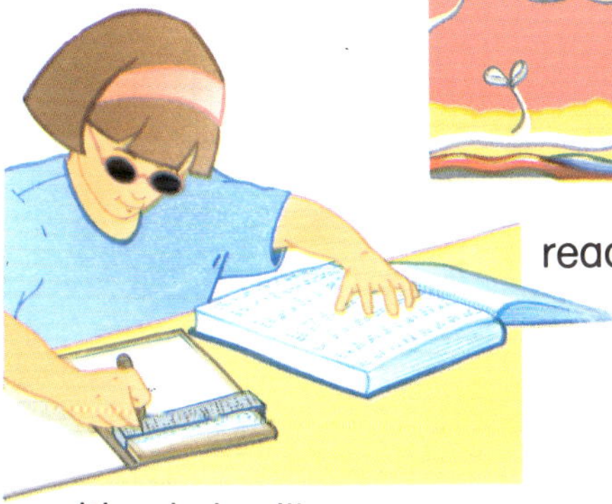

reading in braille

writing in braille

A blind person can read and write braille, by using her sense of touch.

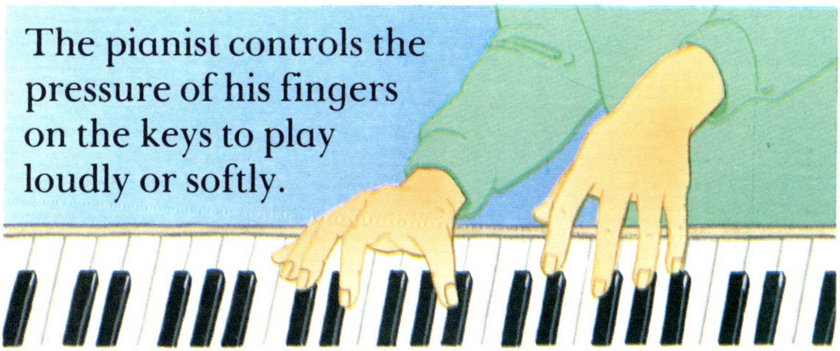

The pianist controls the pressure of his fingers on the keys to play loudly or softly.

Taste

The tongue feels heat and cold, pain and different tastes.

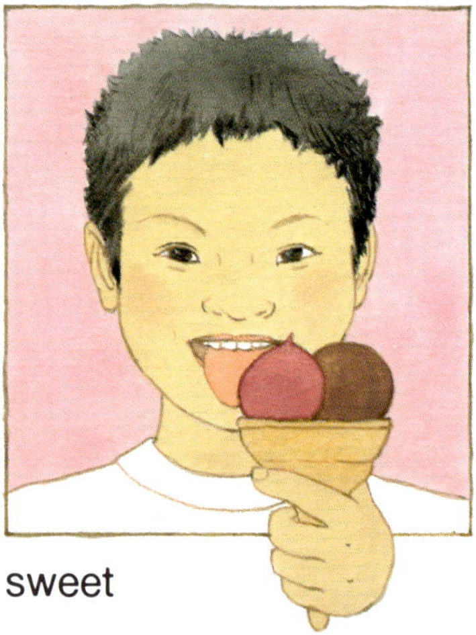

sweet

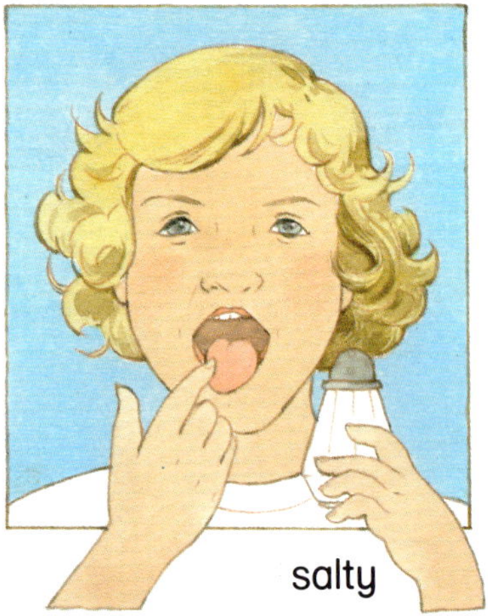

salty

There are thousands of little bumps called taste buds all over your tongue. Inside the buds are nerves that send messages to the brain about what you are eating.

There are four types of taste: sweet, salty, bitter and sour. The tongue has areas which are especially good at recognizing each one of these tastes.

The best way to taste ice cream is to lick it with the tip of your tongue, which is the best part for picking up sweet tastes.

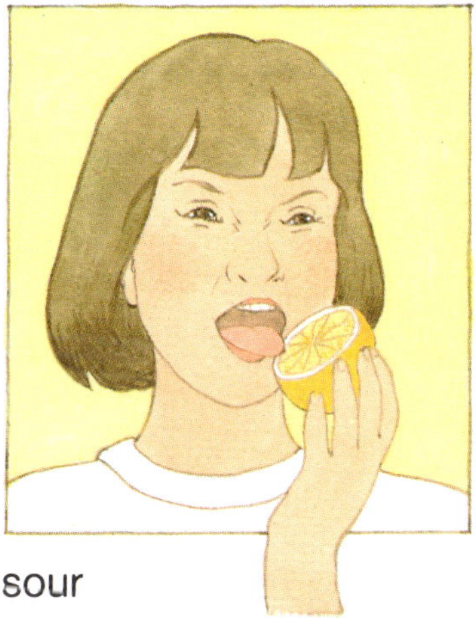

sour

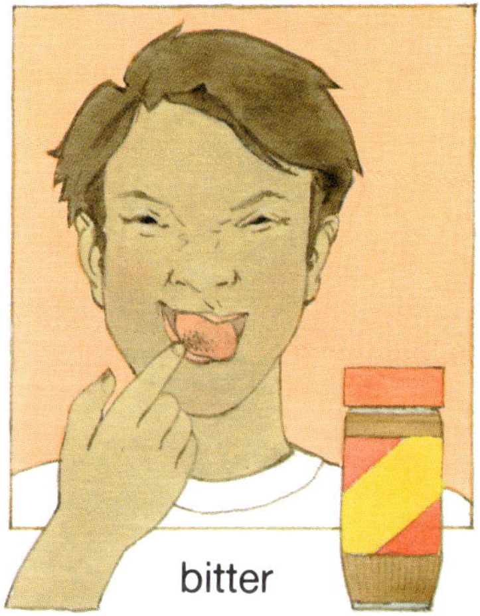

bitter

The back of the tongue recognizes bitter tastes.

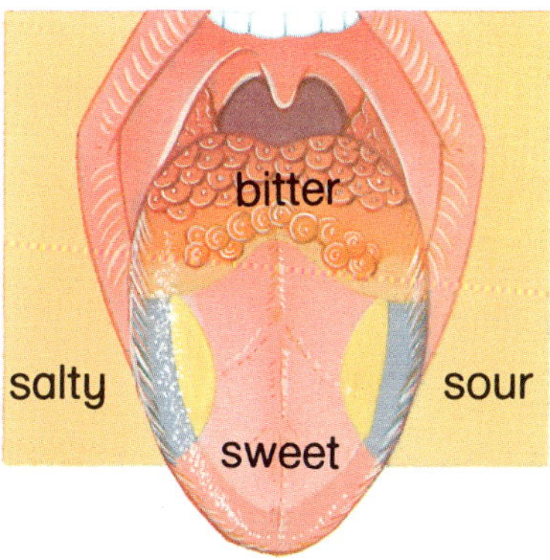

The sides recognize sour and salty tastes.

The front recognizes sweet tastes.

Sight

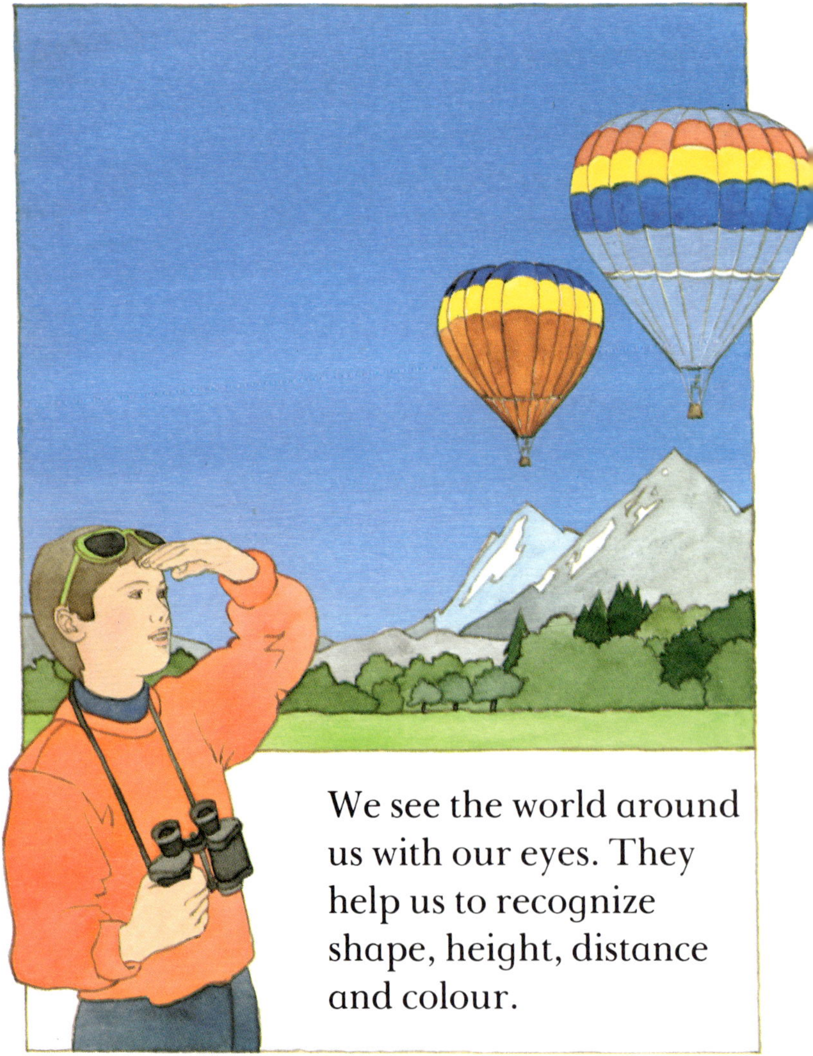

We see the world around us with our eyes. They help us to recognize shape, height, distance and colour.

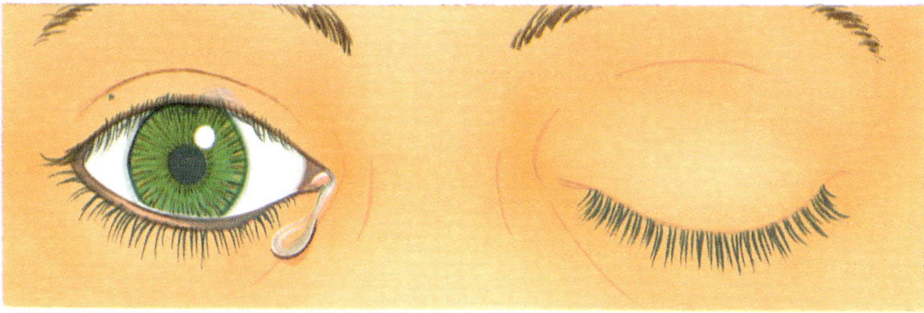

Every time you blink, your eyelids spread tears over your eyes, to keep them moist and clean.

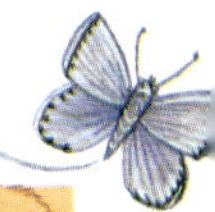

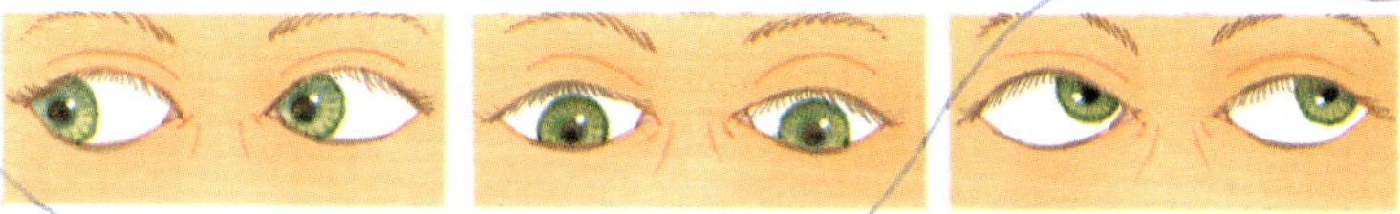

The eye is shaped like a ball. It has muscles attached to it, so it can move up and down and side to side.

Light bounces off the things you look at and enters your eye through the pupil. Nerves in the retina send messages to the brain. The brain tells you what you see.

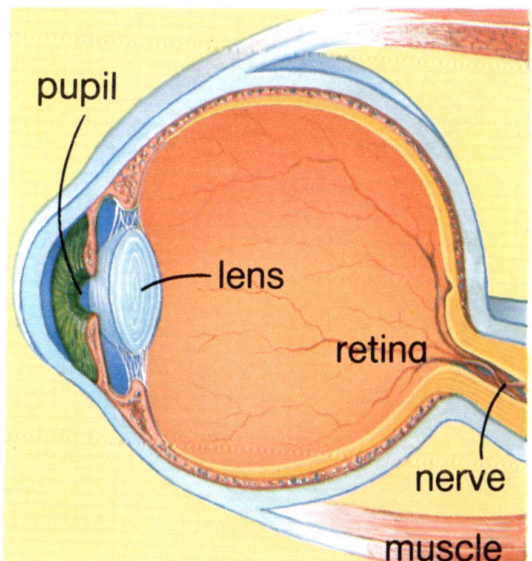

The eyes

When it is dark your pupils grow larger, to let in more light. This helps you see better.

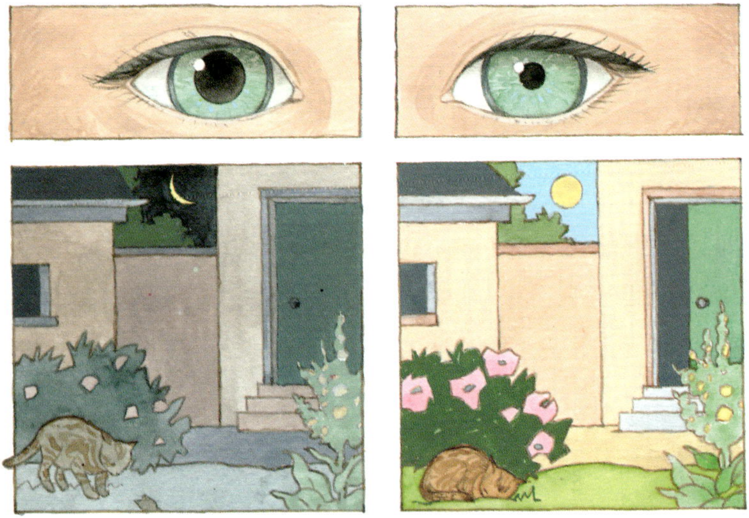

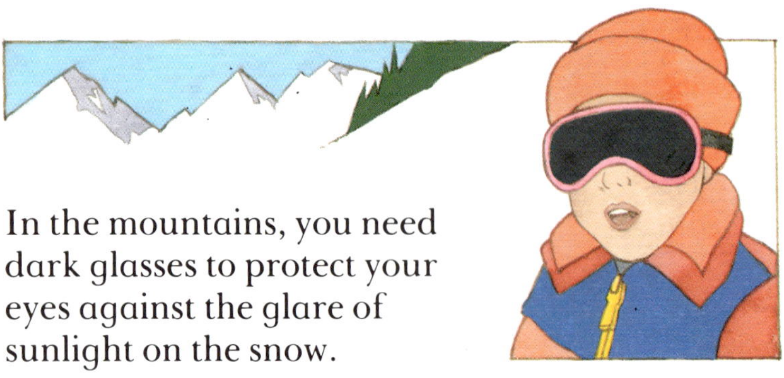

In the mountains, you need dark glasses to protect your eyes against the glare of sunlight on the snow.

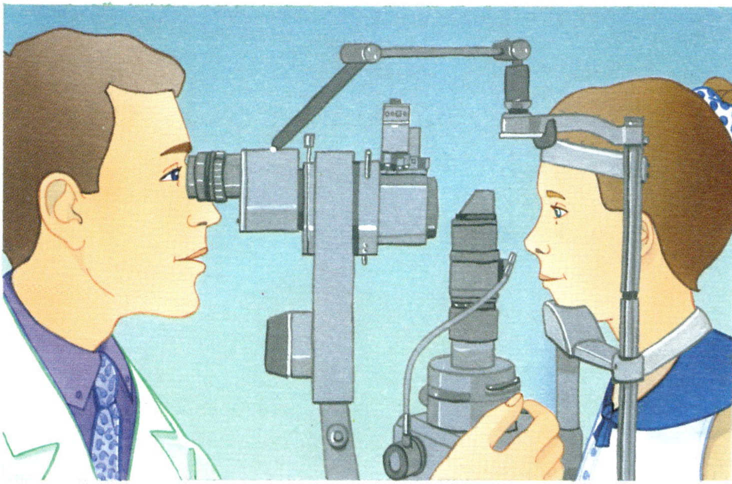

The optician examines eyes with a special instrument. He sees through the pupil to the retina at the back of the eye.

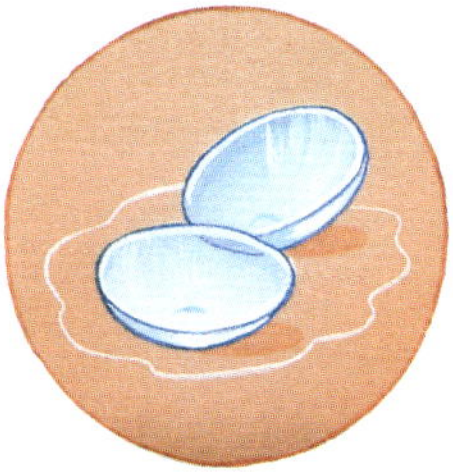

Not everyone can see well. Some people wear glasses or contact lenses to improve their eyesight.

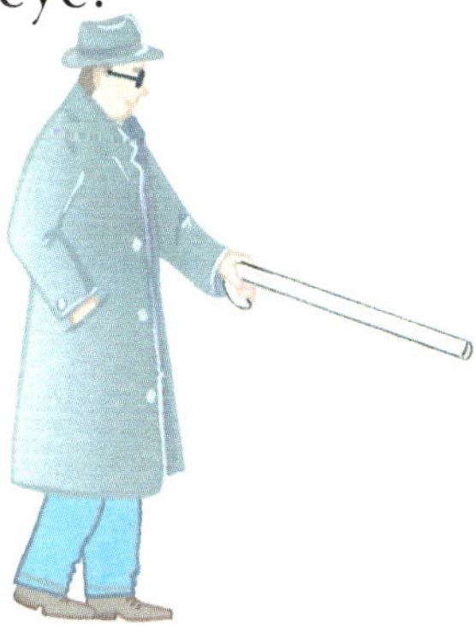

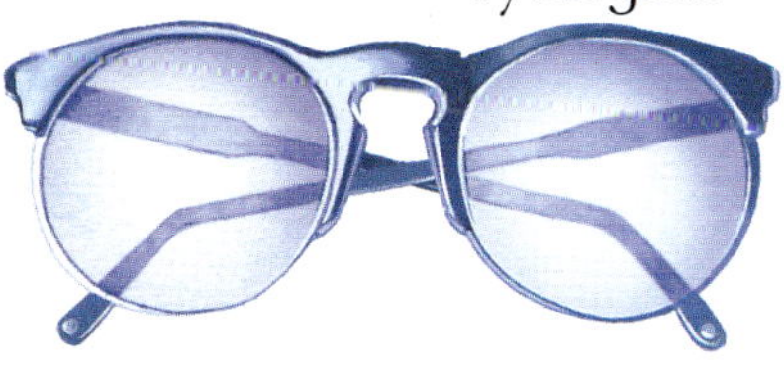

Blind people find their way with a white stick.

The voice

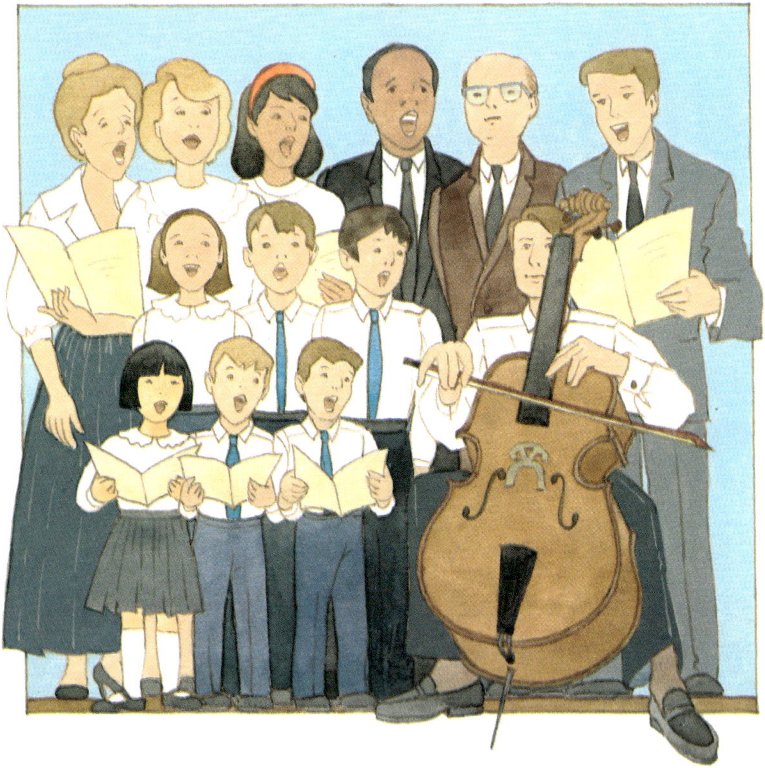

We can talk, shout, laugh and sing. The sounds are made by vocal cords in our throats. We form words by moving our tongue, lips and jaws.

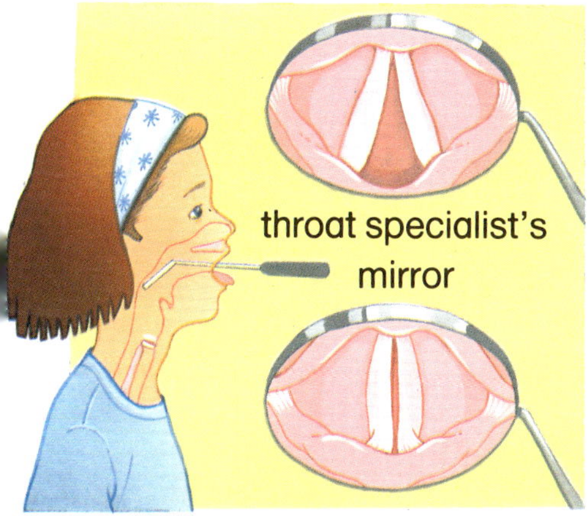

Our vocal cords are two stretchy flaps. The air we breathe out makes them vibrate. This is what produces sounds.

The harder we breathe out, the louder our voice is. If you put your fingers on your throat while you sing, you can feel the vibrations.

Some people cannot speak. They use sign language instead.

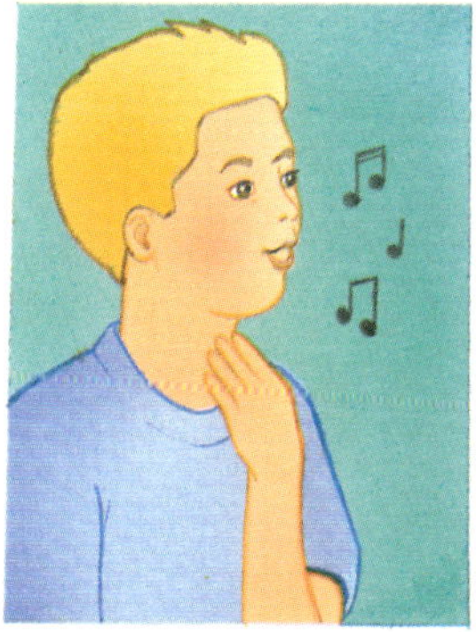

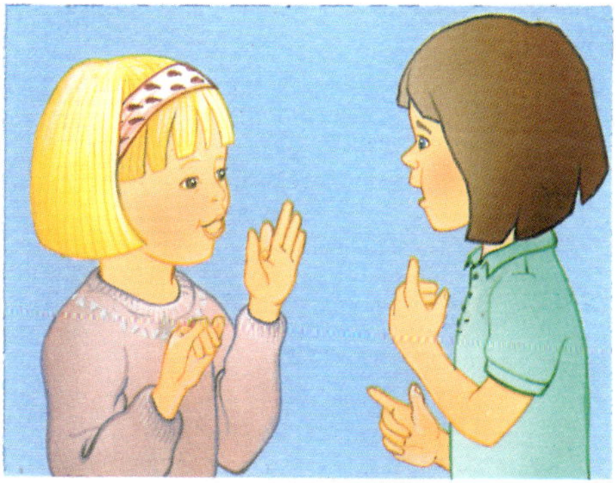

Body talk

The body has a silent language of its own. It can express our feelings without words.

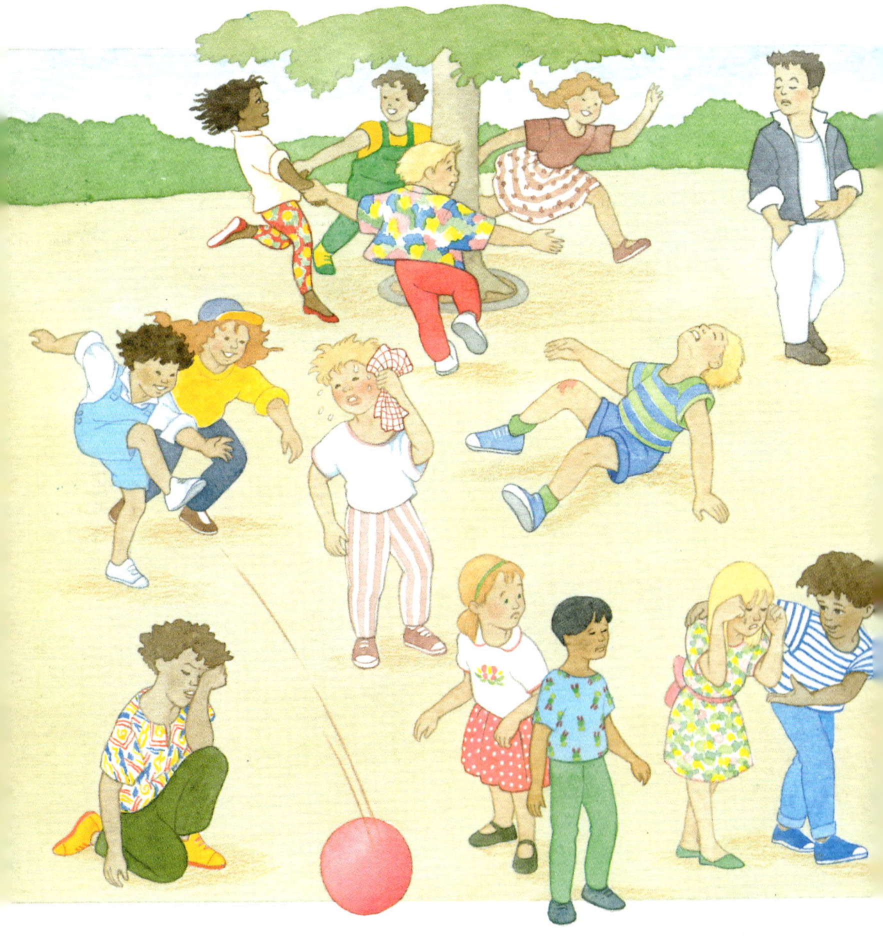

The way people stand, the gestures they make with their hands, and the expressions on their faces all send clear messages. When we are happy, we look different from when we are sad.

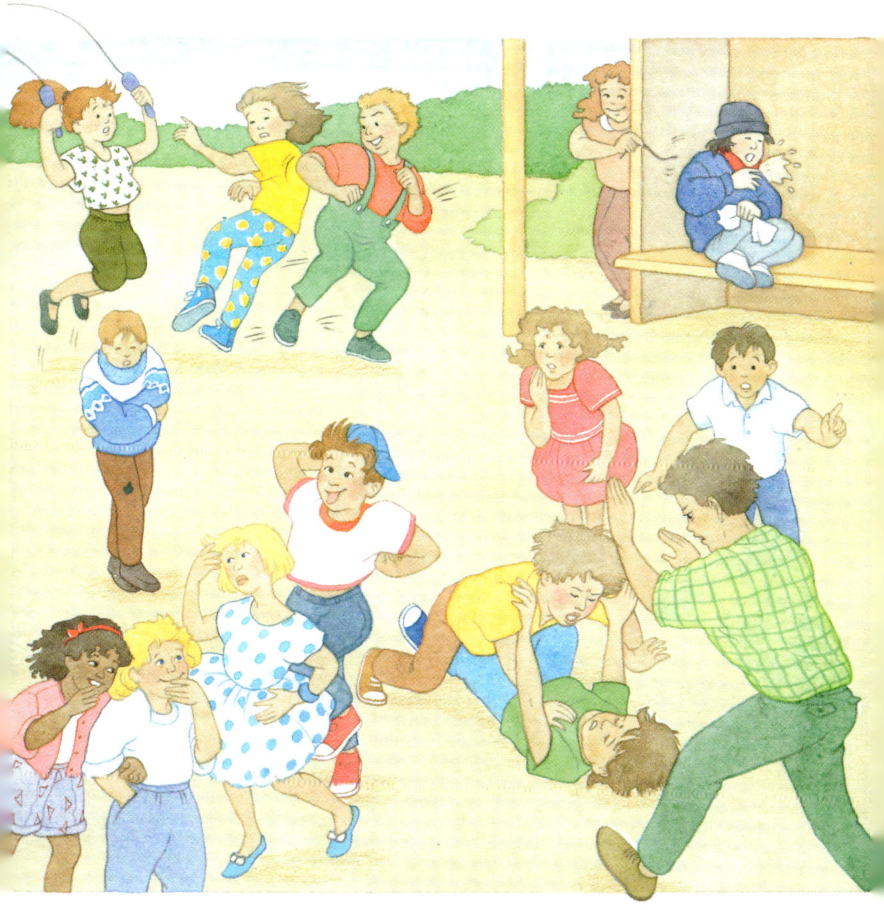

When you are ill

When we are ill, we may have a high temperature, a cough, spots, or aches and pains. These are signs that the body is being attacked by germs.

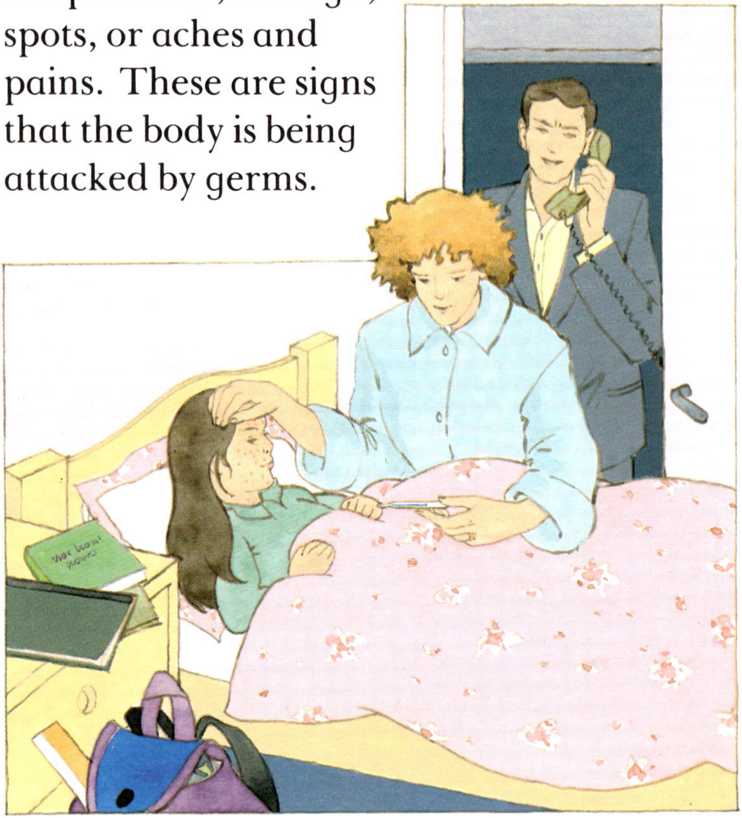

When the body is fighting off invading germs, it works harder and the heart beats faster. The body's temperature rises.

The doctor examines you to find out which part of you the germs are attacking. She listens to your heart and lungs with a stethoscope, looks in your ears and throat, and asks you questions. Then the doctor decides if you need anything to help you get better.

You may need medicine to fight against the germs.

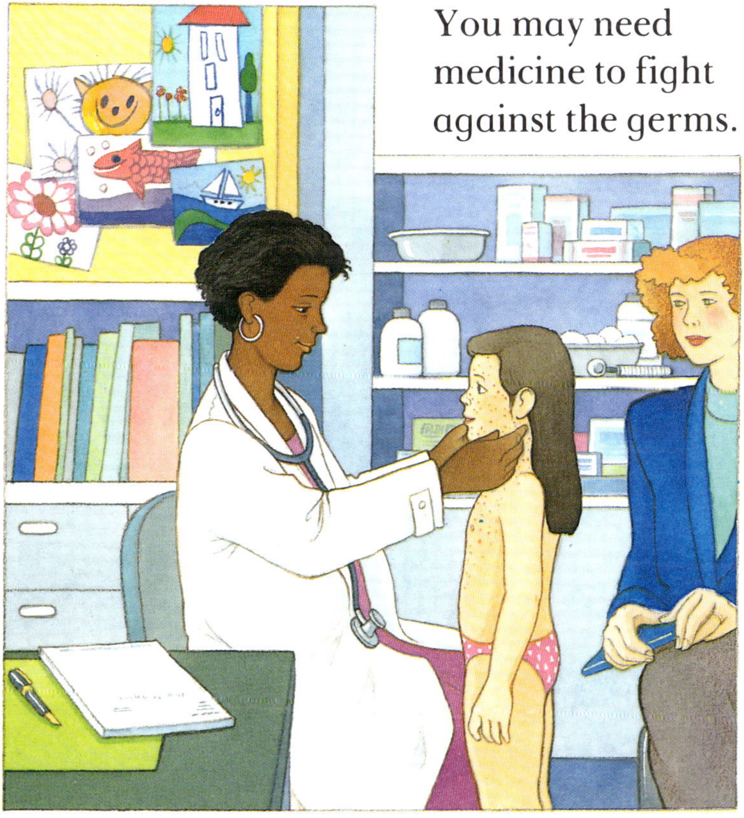

Out of danger

Diseases such as chickenpox are very catching. But you catch some of them only once. After that, the body recognizes the disease and protects itself against it.

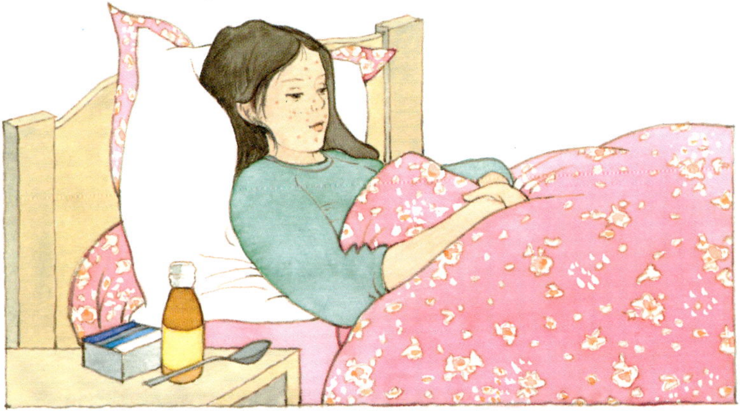

So you can visit a friend who has chickenpox if you have already had it.

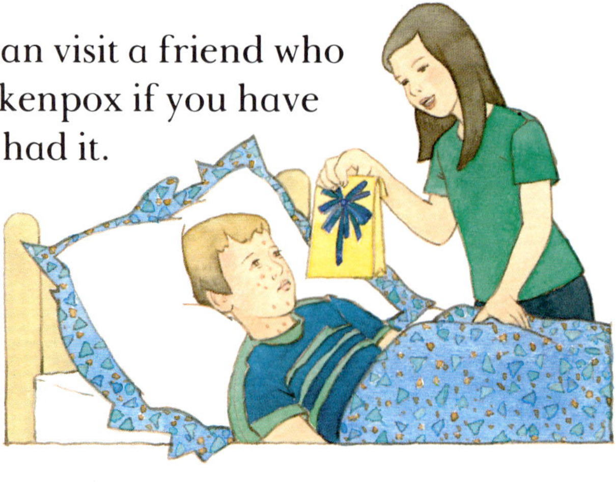

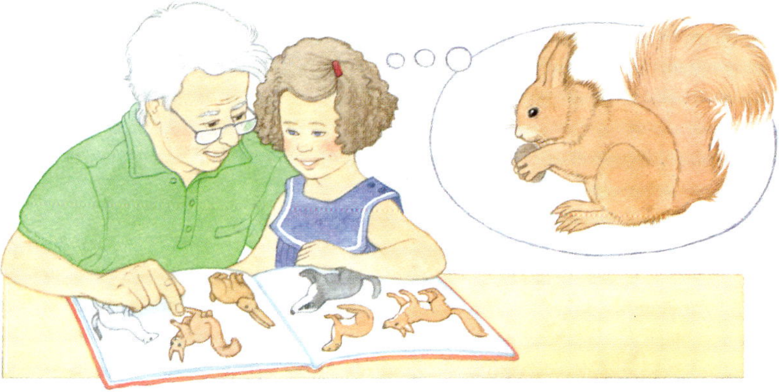

The brain stores information. This is called memory. It is what helps you to talk, learn and think.

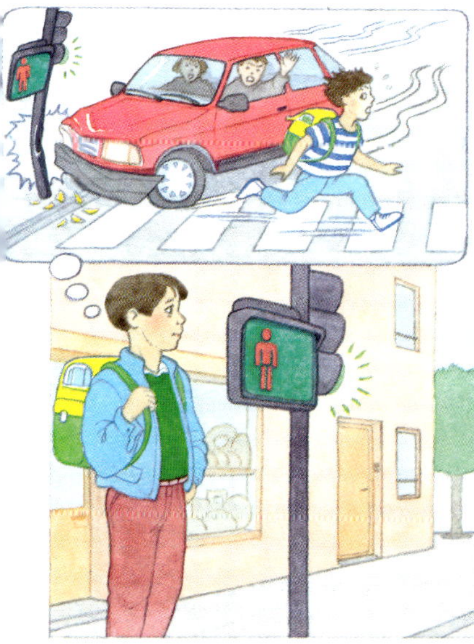

The brain helps us to avoid accidents. We remember to take care when we cross the road.

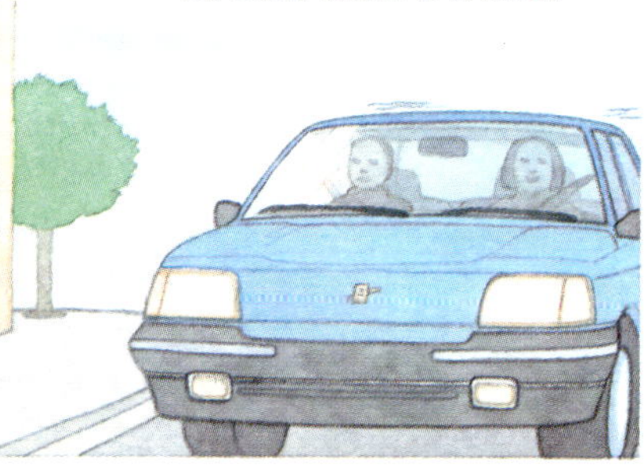

Amazing facts

Your ears help you to keep your balance. When you move, liquid in your ear moves and sets off nerves that tell your brain about the position of your body.

Fingertips are very sensitive. The skin there has more nerve endings than the skin on other parts of the body.

Some people are colour-blind. This means they confuse colours. For example, they may think green is red and red is green.

People mostly rely on sight to find things. Dogs use their noses more. Bats hunt at night, so they need to hear well.

A voice can be so high-pitched that its sound cracks a crystal glass!

The systems

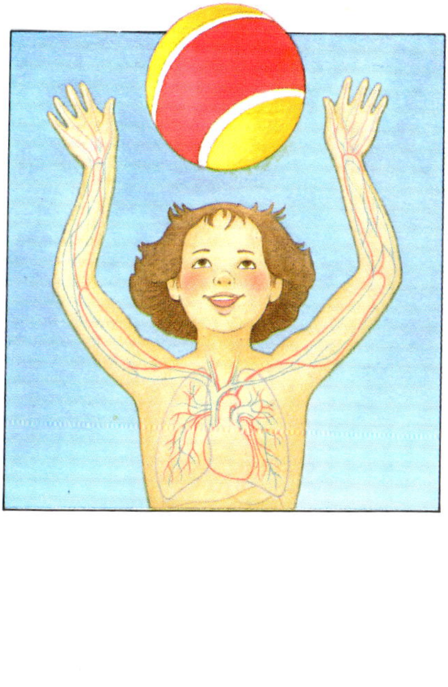

Eating for energy

We eat food because it gives our bodies energy. People eat many kinds of food, but our bodies digest everything in the same way.

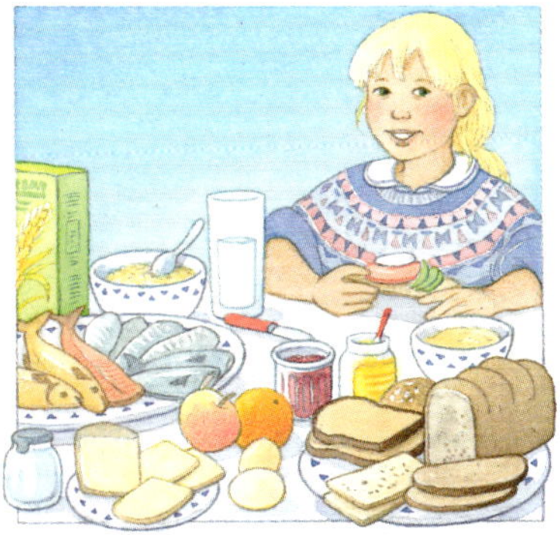

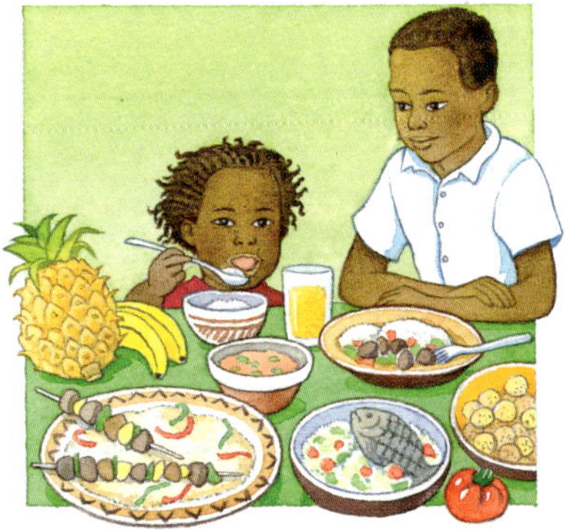

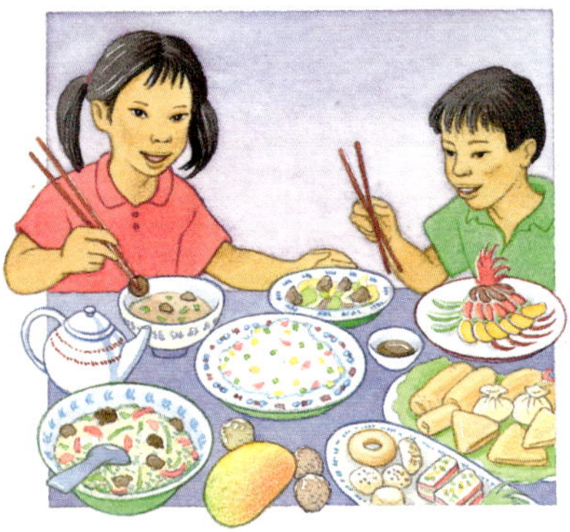

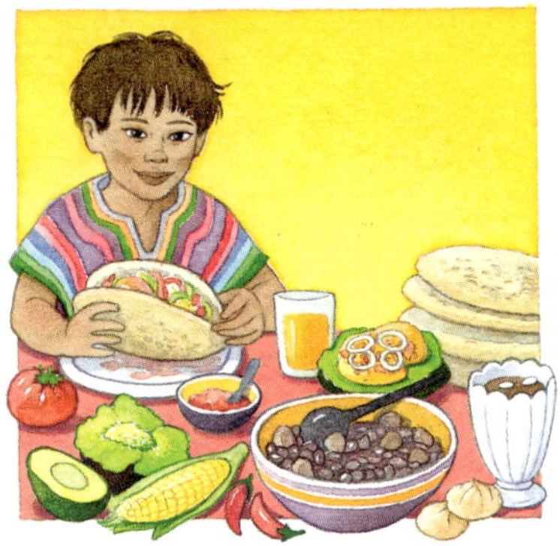

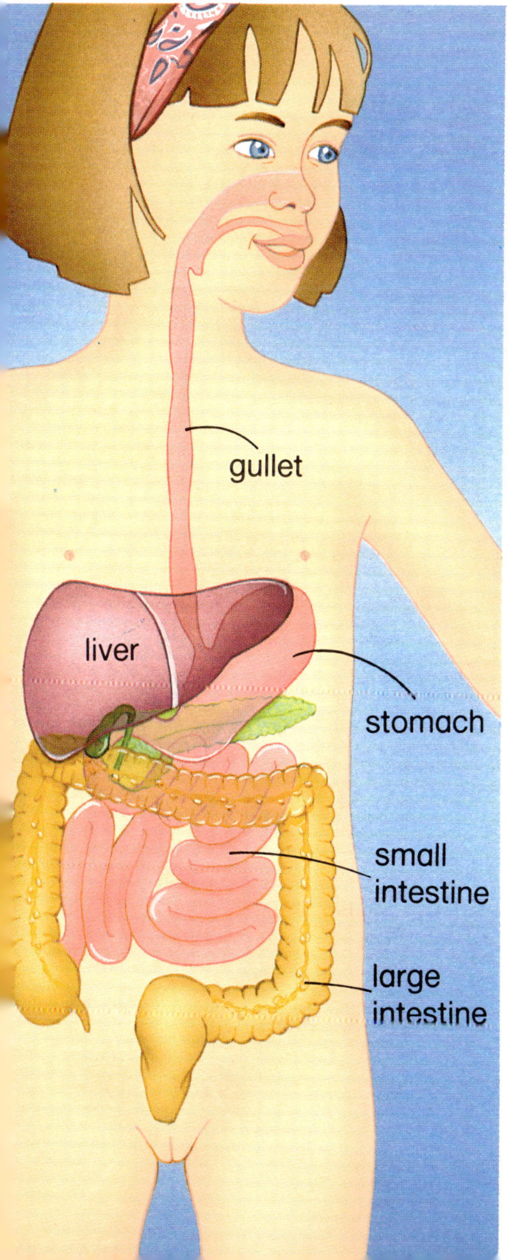

When you swallow food, it moves down a tube into the stomach. The stomach mashes it into pulp. Next, it is squeezed along your intestines.

Now the food is digested, and it passes through the intestine into the blood. The blood takes it around your body.

Thc body gets rid of the food it cannot use when we go to the lavatory.

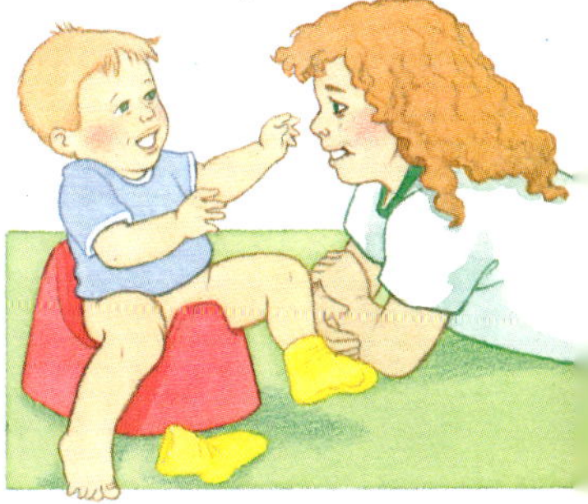

Teeth

We bite into food and chew it with our teeth so it is easier to swallow and digest. The sharp incisors at the front are for cutting. Pointed canines at the sides are for tearing. Big molars at the back are for crushing.

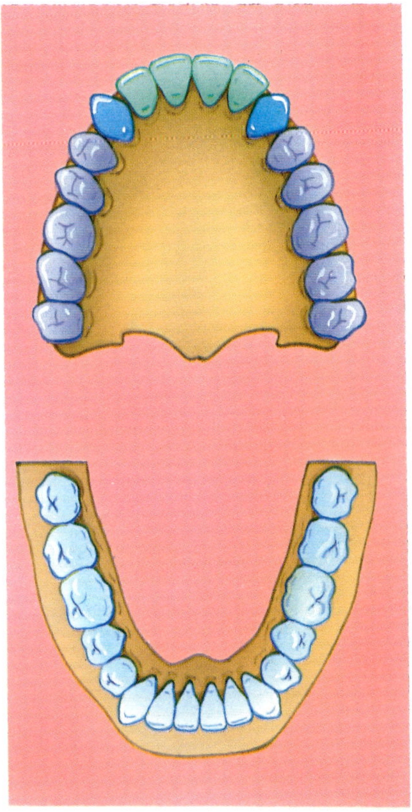

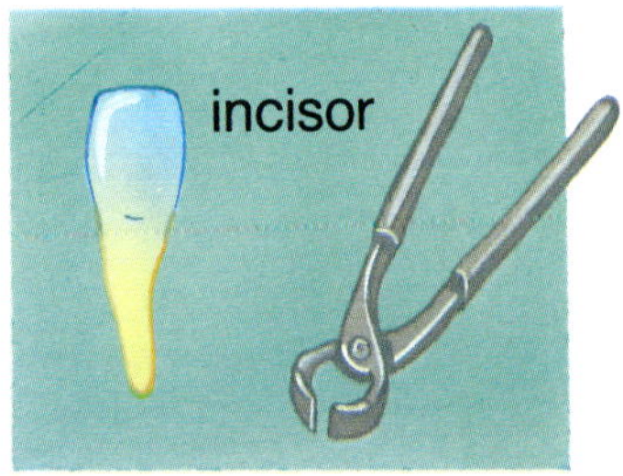

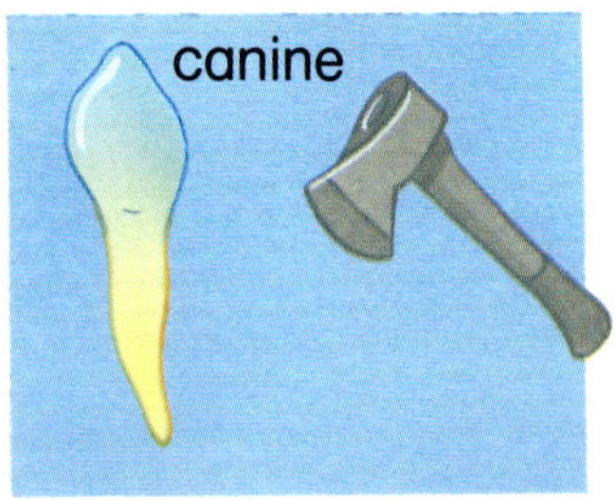

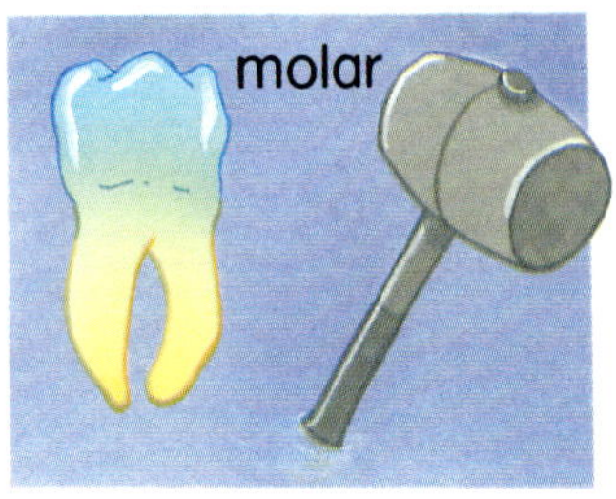

A hard layer of enamel covers the dentine. Inside this is the pulp, the sensitive part. Under the gum, each tooth has a root that holds it in place in the jaw bone.

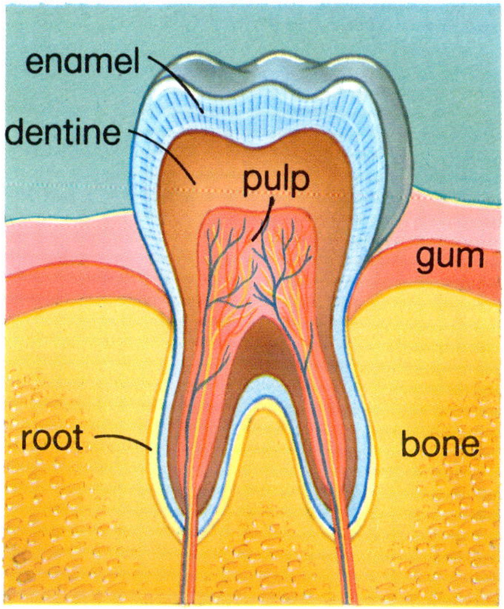

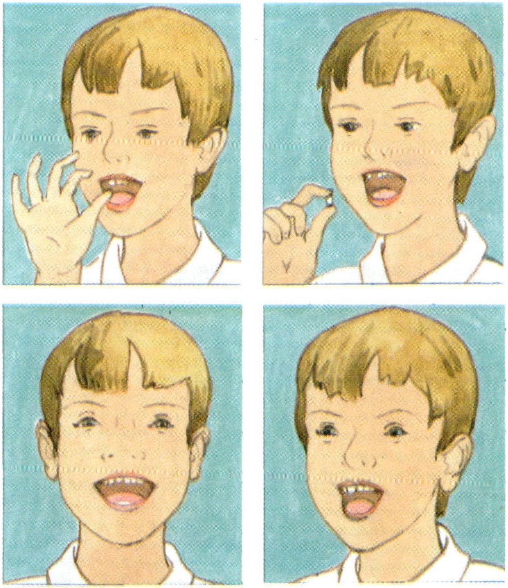

When we are about six years old, our first teeth become loose and fall out.

They make room for the larger teeth that are growing underneath.

At the dentist's

The dentist looks after our teeth. If he finds a decaying tooth with a hole, he removes the decay and fills the hole with hard paste.

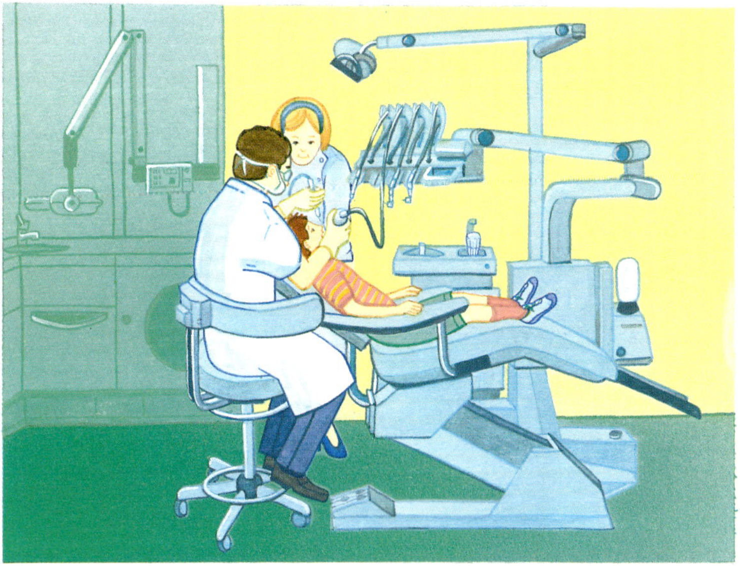

Crooked teeth can be straightened by wearing a brace or plate.

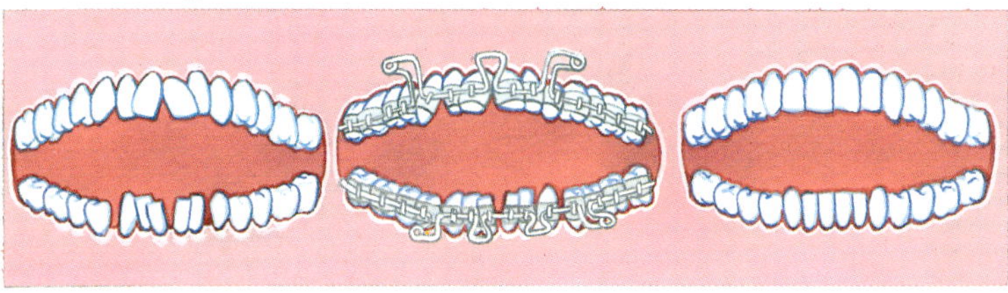

Brushing your teeth for three minutes twice a day helps to prevent decay.

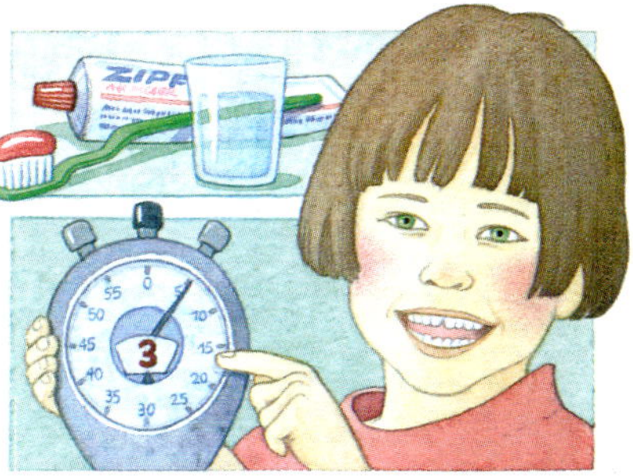

When you brush your teeth, you get rid of the food scraps and germs that cause decay.

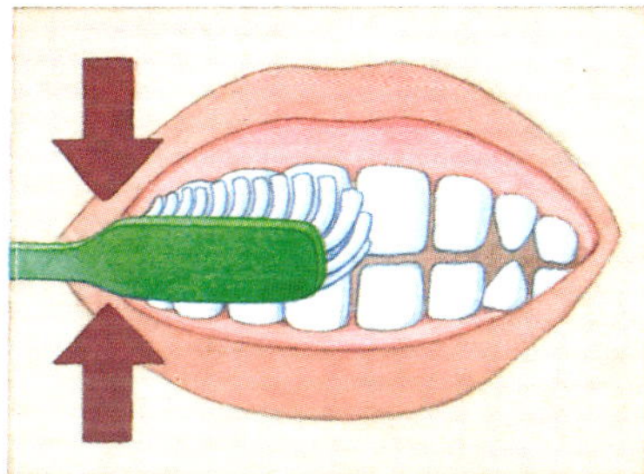

Always brush from pink to white, from the gums to the teeth.

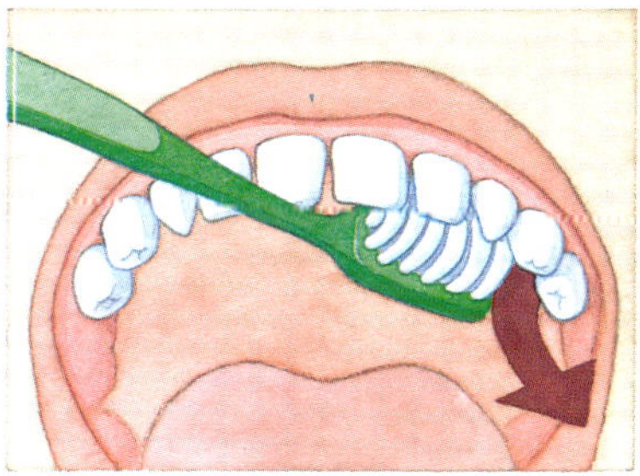

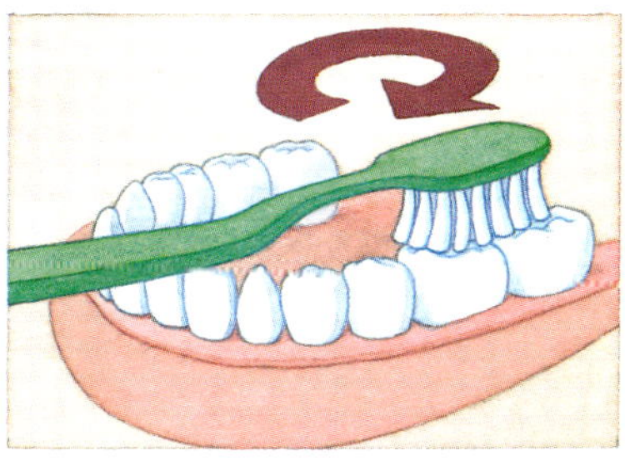

The heart

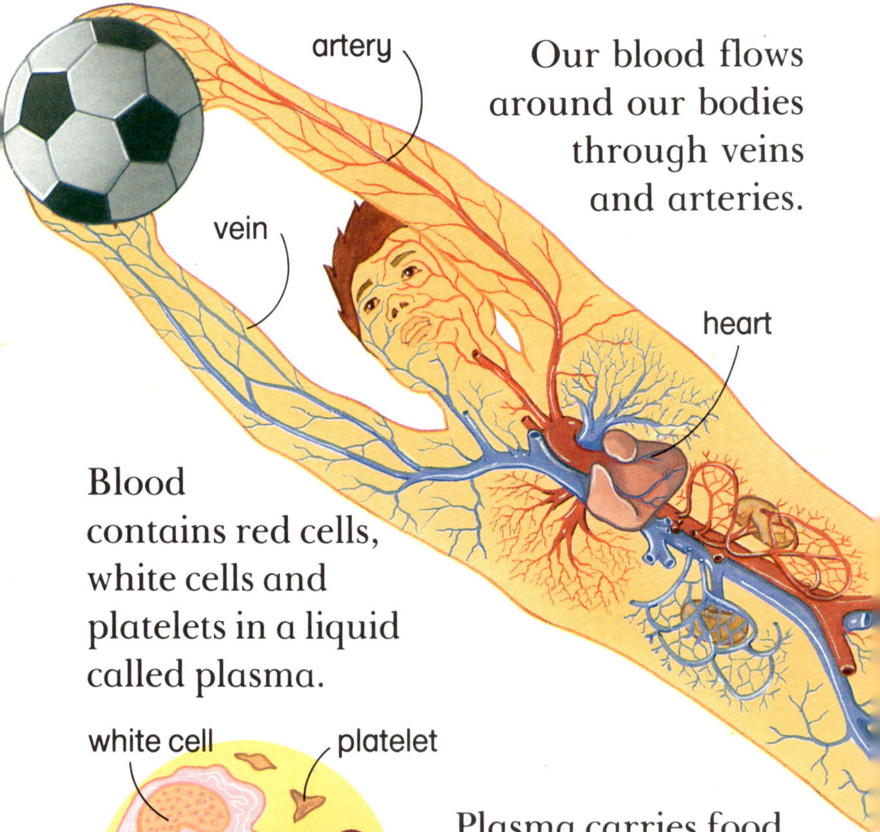

Our blood flows around our bodies through veins and arteries.

Blood contains red cells, white cells and platelets in a liquid called plasma.

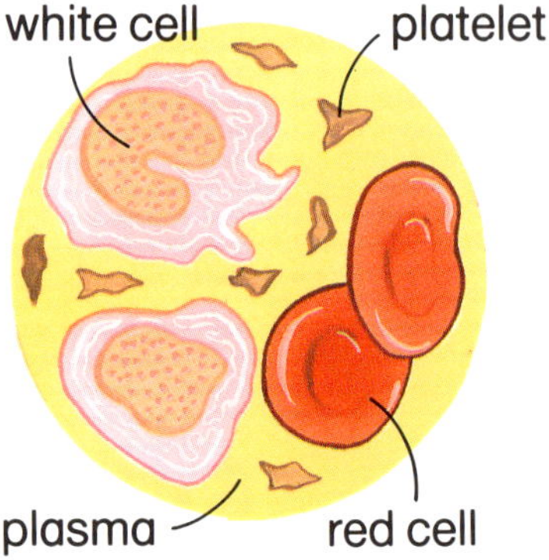

Plasma carries food to the body's cells. Red cells carry oxygen. White cells kill germs. Platelets help to stop bleeding.

The heart is a hollow muscle. As it contracts or beats, it pumps blood around the body.

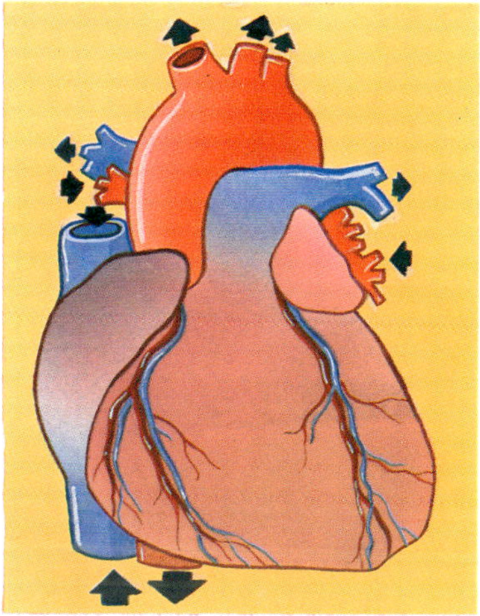

Your heart works all day and all night, without stopping.

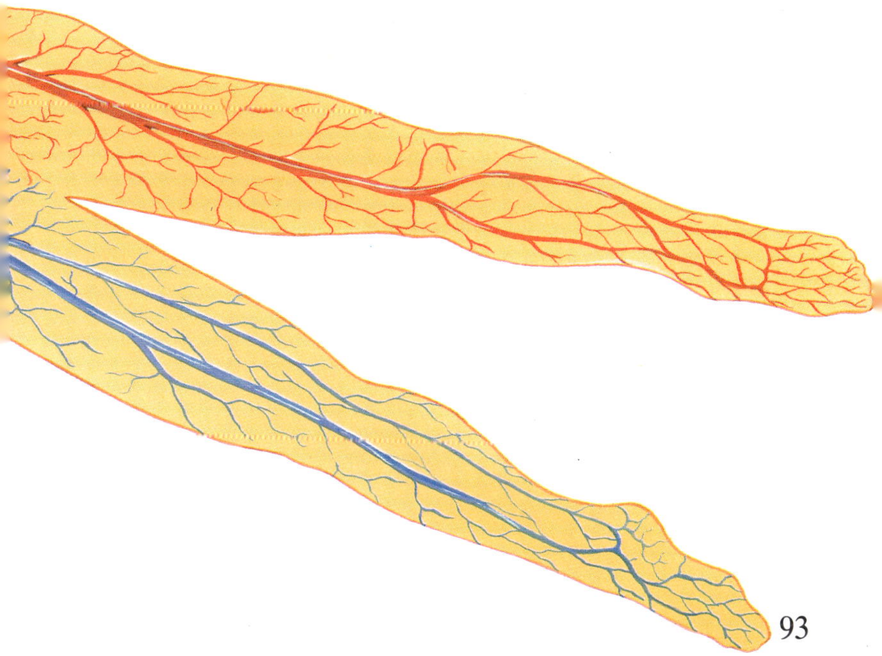

Breathing

We need oxygen to stay alive. Our lungs take oxygen from the air we breathe. Our blood takes the oxygen from the lungs and carries it to the rest of the body.

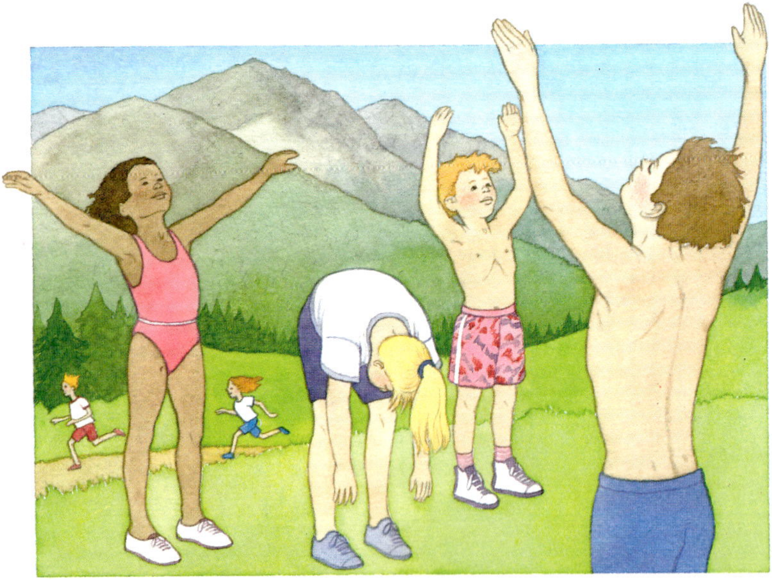

It is impossible to stay under water without a snorkel or air tanks, because there is no air to breathe.

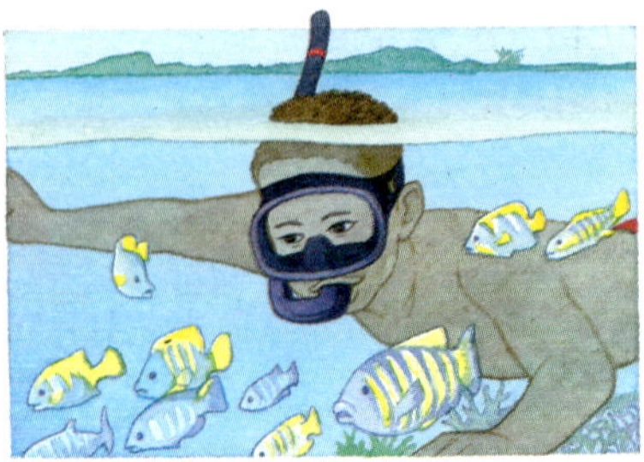

When you breathe in through your nose or your mouth, air goes down your windpipe and into your lungs.

Blood travels through your lungs and collects oxygen from them. Blood also carries used air back to the lungs.

When you breathe out, your lungs push the used air back out through your nose or your mouth.

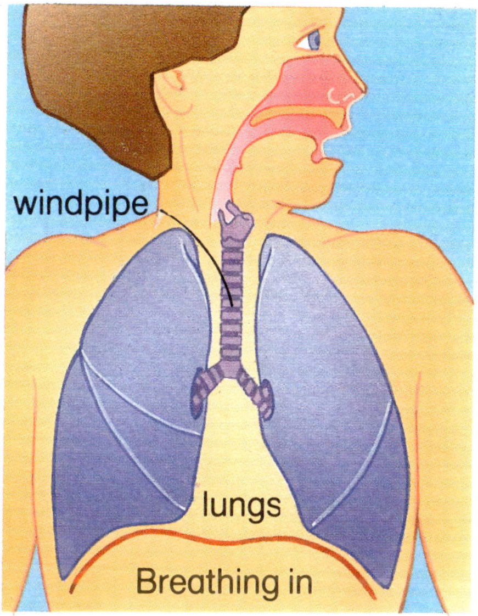

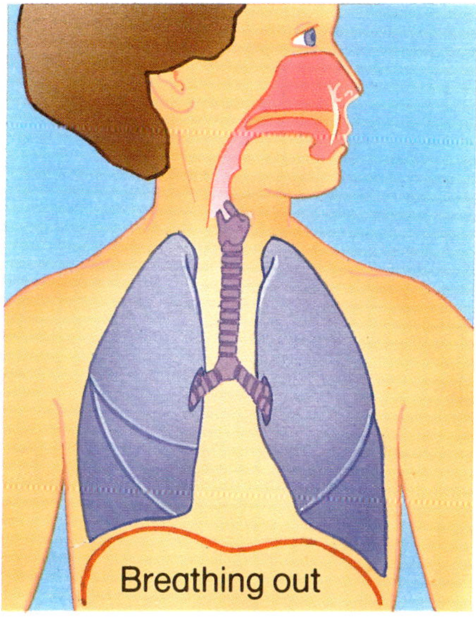

Male and female

Men and women have different organs for making a baby.

A woman has:
- two ovaries that produce an egg each month;
- two tubes that link the ovaries to the womb;
- the womb, where the fertilized egg grows into a baby;
- the vagina.

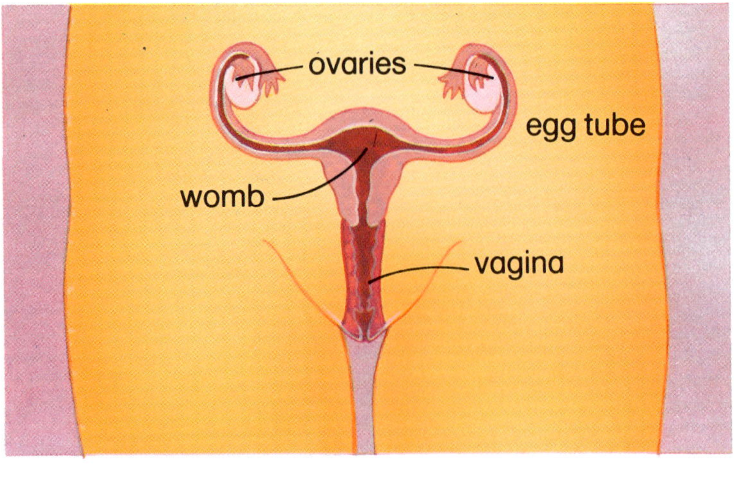

A man has:

- two testicles that make sperm;
- two tubes that pass sperm to the penis;
- the penis.

These organs are ready to make a baby only after adolescence, when we grow into men and women.

You can find out how a baby is made if you turn back to page 46.

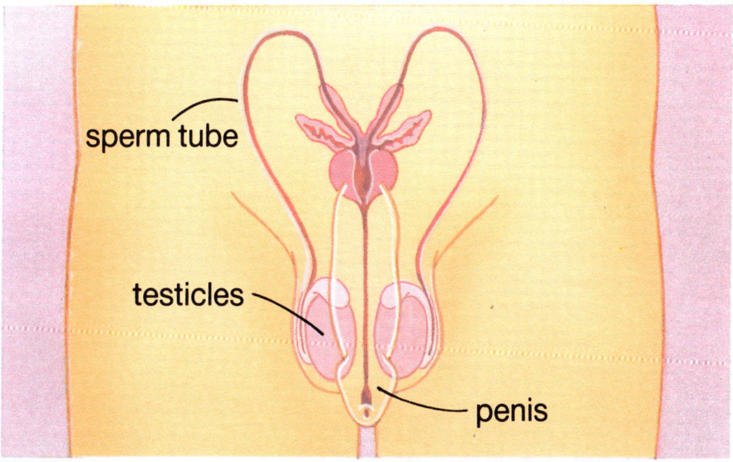

Getting rid of waste

As your body works, it creates waste products. The body gets rid of them in several ways. We breathe out used air. Our sweat gets rid of salt and other waste.

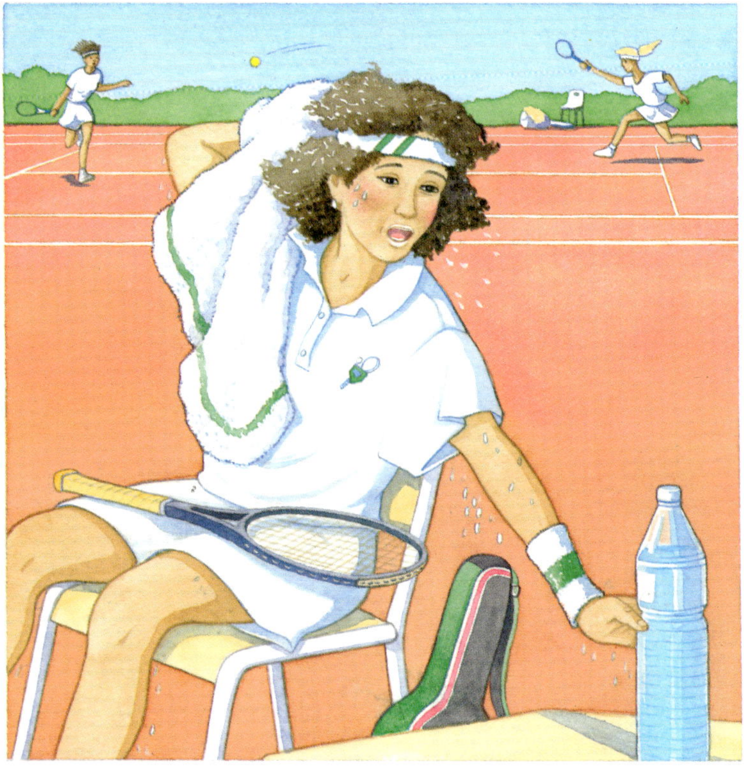

Our kidneys also get rid of waste.

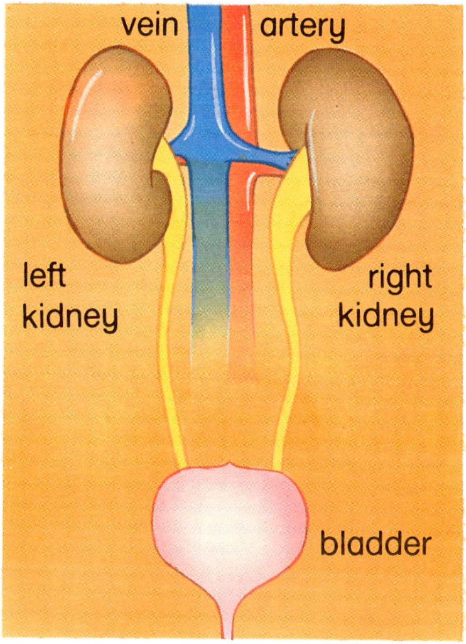

Blood flows through the kidneys. They separate water, salt and other waste from the blood. This waste is turned into urine and stored in a pouch called the bladder.

When the bladder is full, we have to go to the lavatory.

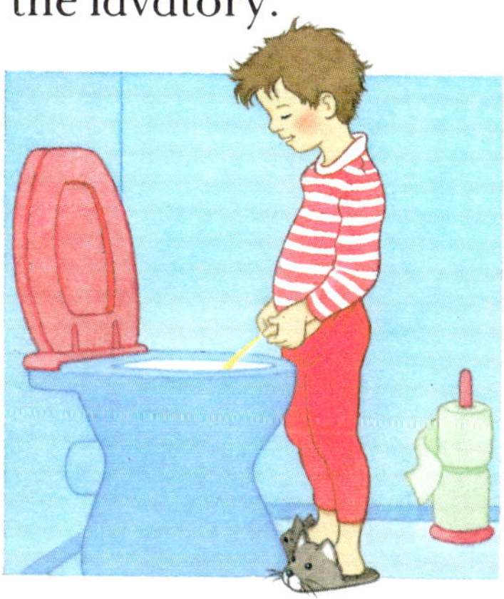

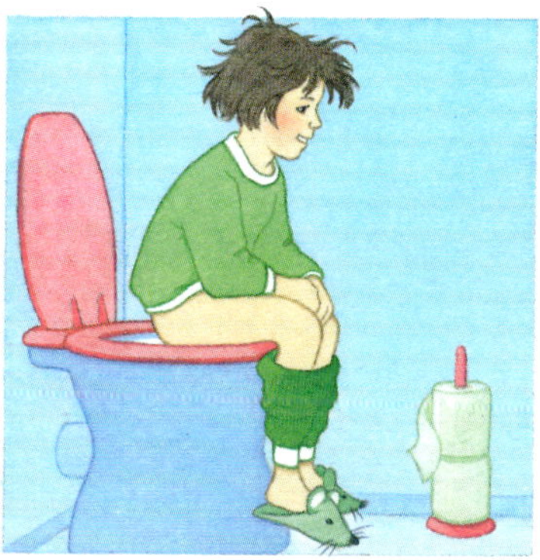

The nervous system

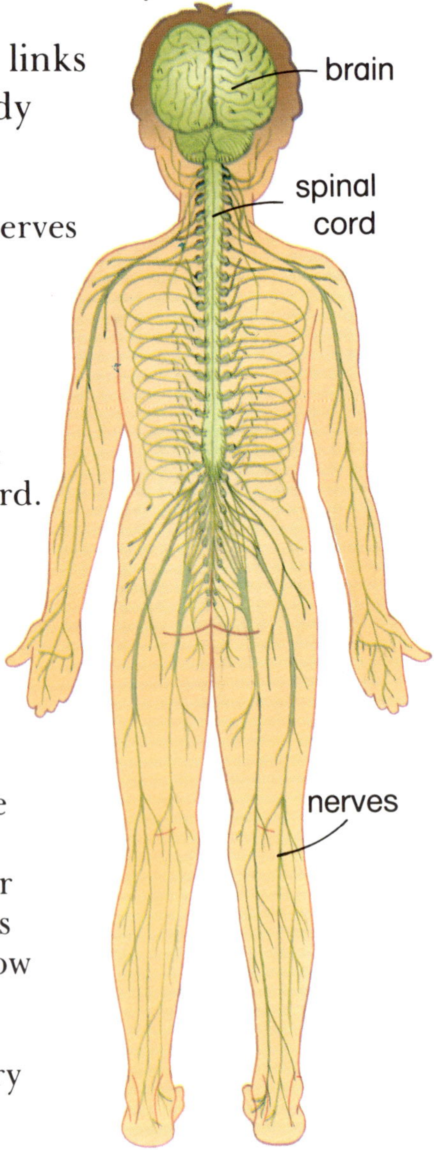

A network of nerves links every part of the body with the brain.

From our senses, the nerves receive information about our bodies and the world around us.

The nerves send the information as electric signals to the spinal cord. This is a thick bundle of nerves down the middle of our backs. The spinal cord carries the signals up to the brain.

The brain sorts out the information. It sends commands along other nerves to tell the body's organs and muscles how to react.

All of this happens very quickly, in less than a second.

Our nervous system helps us to use our senses, to think, remember and plan, and to move.

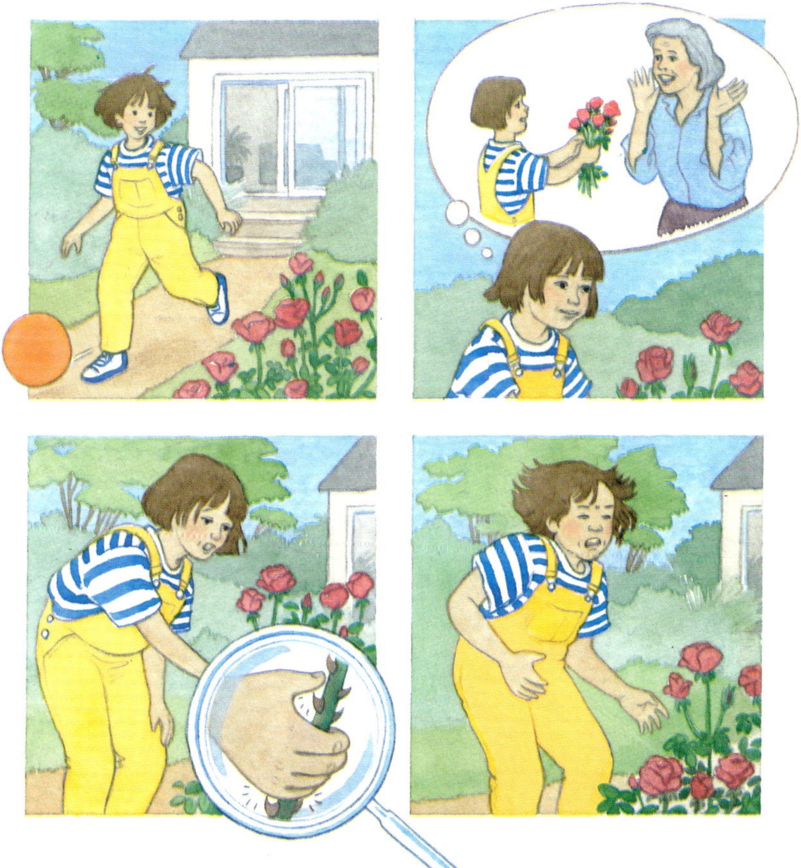

Sometimes we do things without thinking. When you touch something sharp, your hand will jerk away, without waiting for a message from the brain. This is called reflex action.

Amazing facts

- As we grow up, we have more blood. A new-born baby has less than half a litre of blood, an eight year old has about 1.75 litres and adults have between 5 and 6 litres.

- It takes about one minute for blood to flow from the heart to your toes and back again. To pump blood around your body, your heart beats about 70 times per minute. An elephant's heart beats only 25 times per minute. A mouse's heart beats 500 times per minute.

- You take about 23,000 breaths each day.

- When you sneeze, air rushes out of your nose at about 160 kilometres per hour.

- The fastest nerve signals travel at 400 kilometres per hour. That is about the same speed as a racing car.

Keeping

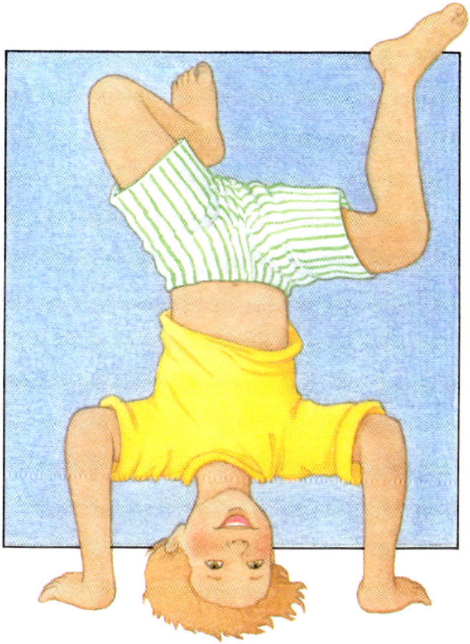

fit

☺ Sleep

While you are asleep, your body keeps working, like a town at night.

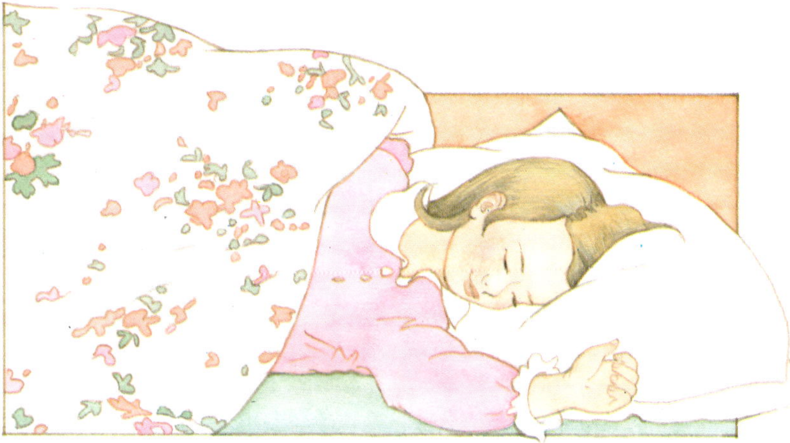

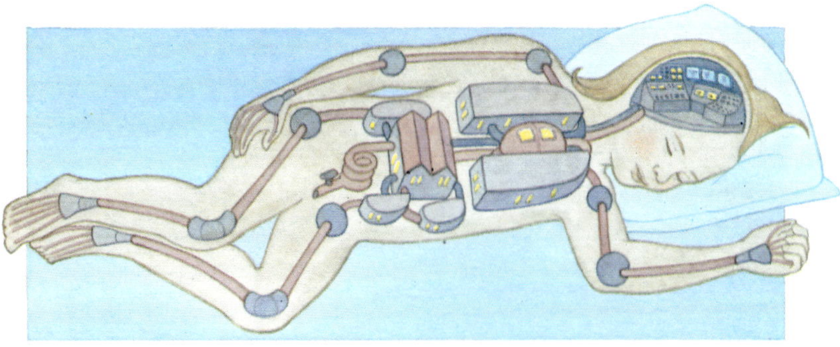

But it works more slowly, so that it can rest and grow.

Most children sleep for about twelve hours every night. Babies need more sleep, and adults need less.

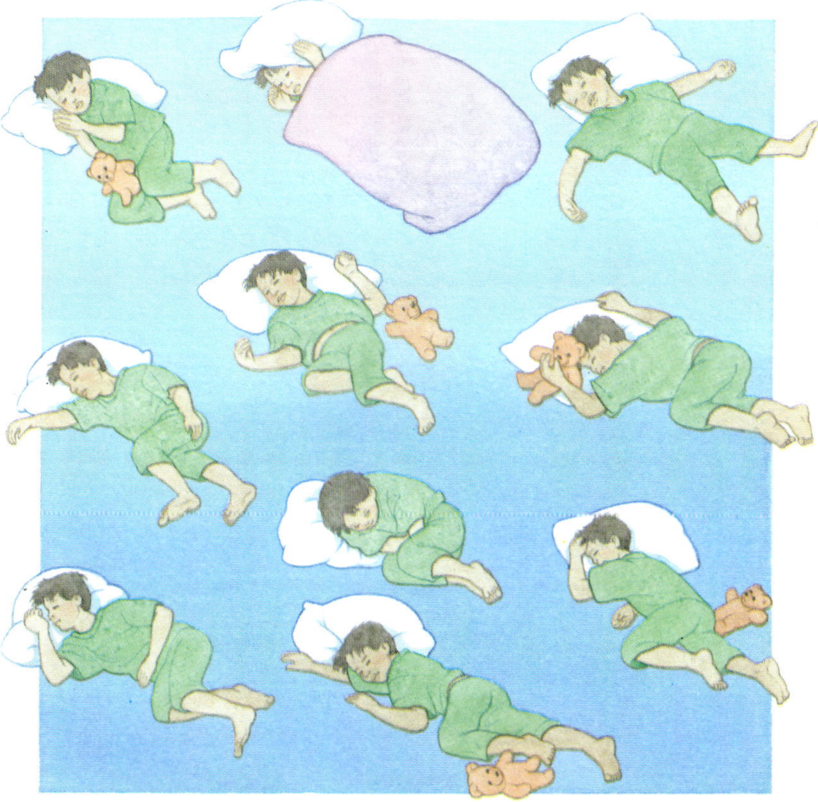

You do not lie completely still all night. You change position many times.

☺ Dreams and nightmares

While we are asleep we have dreams. The stories in our dreams seem real while we are asleep. But we don't always remember them when we wake up.

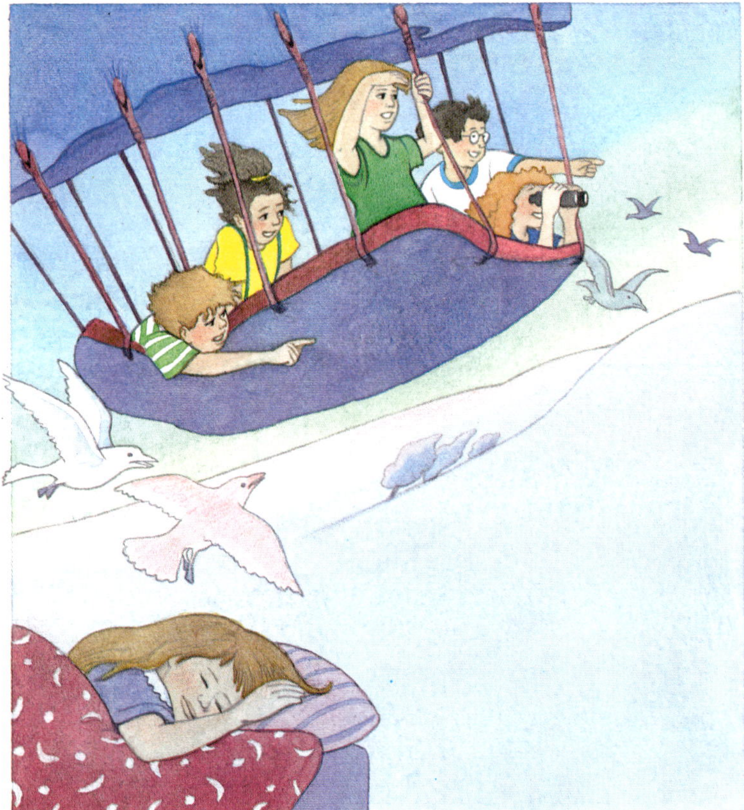

Nightmares are frightening dreams.
Some nightmares are so frightening that they wake us up.
But nightmares are useful because they use up some of the unhappiness and worries we have in real life.

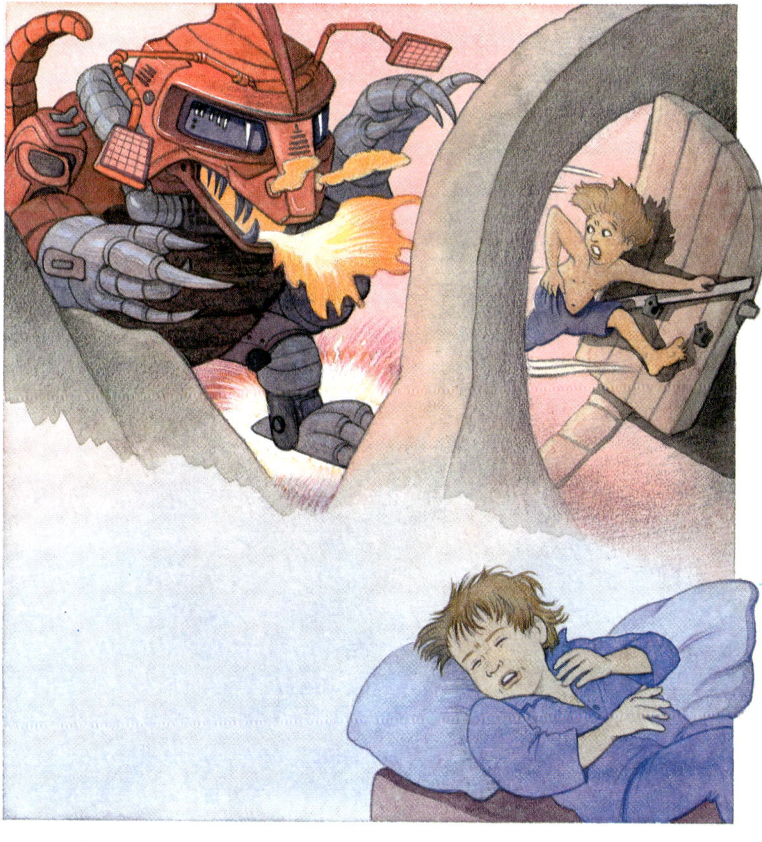

☺ Playing games

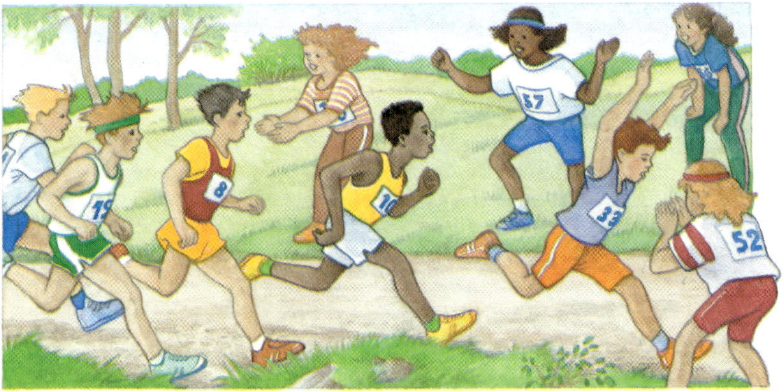

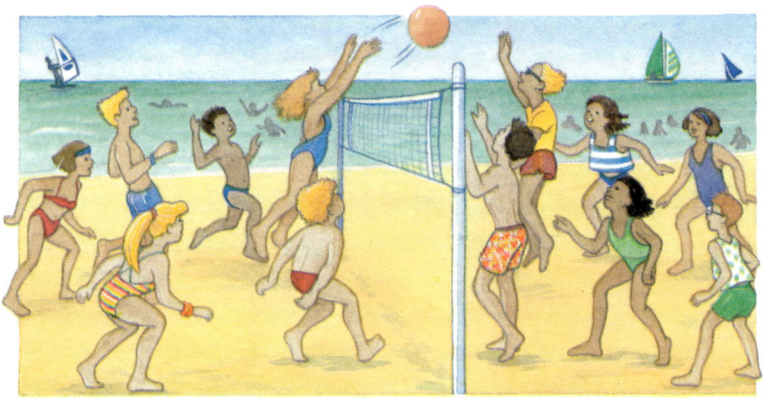

We make full use of our bodies when we play games. Physical exercise helps us to grow stronger. With regular exercise, our bodies become fitter and less easily tired.

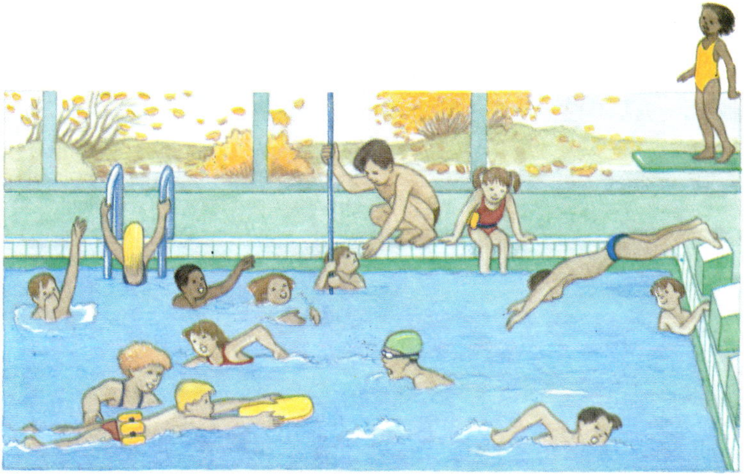

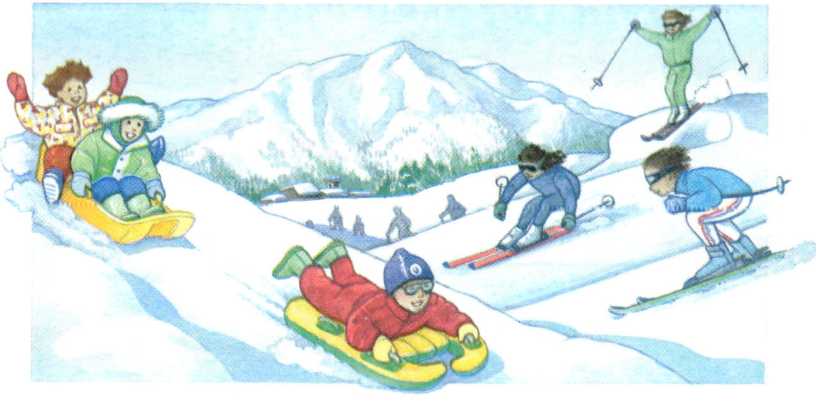

Sports are fun. Whichever sport we choose, we have to follow the rules and concentrate to do well. On our own or in a team, we should play so that everybody has fun.

☺ Healthy meals

Your food should give your body what it needs to keep working. There are three main groups of food. You can help your body by eating food from each group, and by drinking enough water.

These are the three groups. Each type of food acts on the body in a particular way.

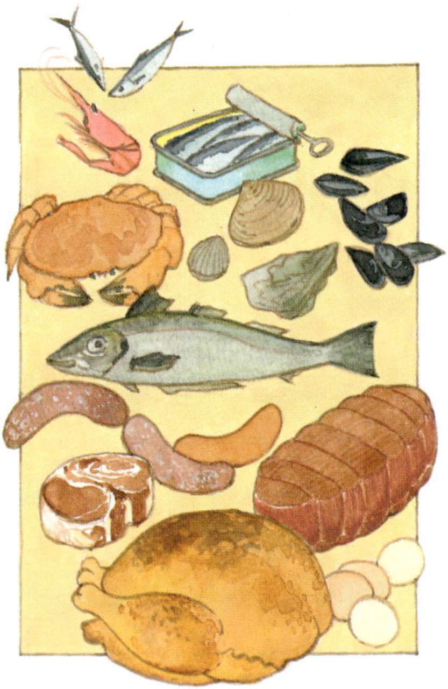

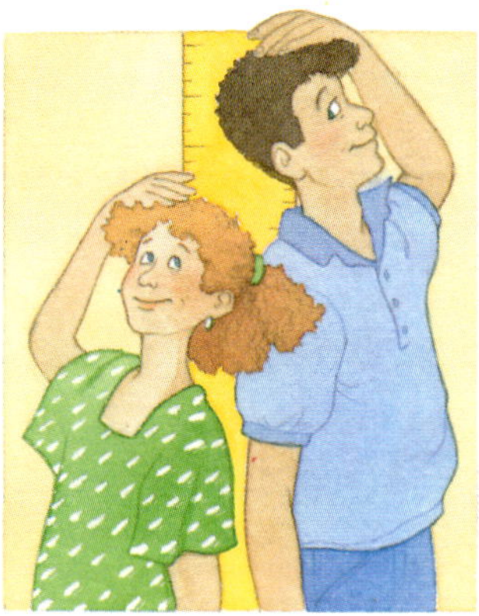

Proteins build and repair cells so that the body can grow and stay strong.

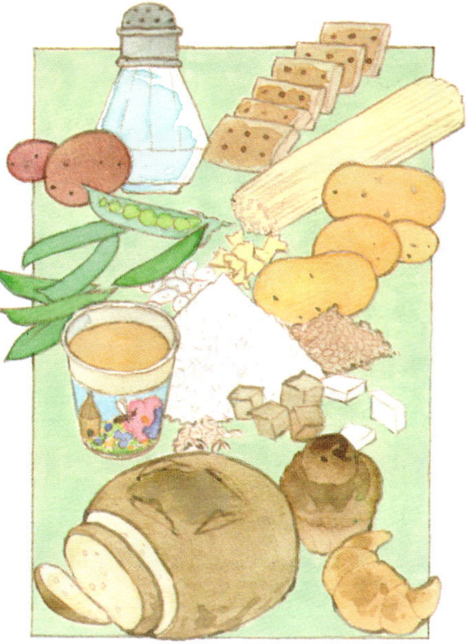

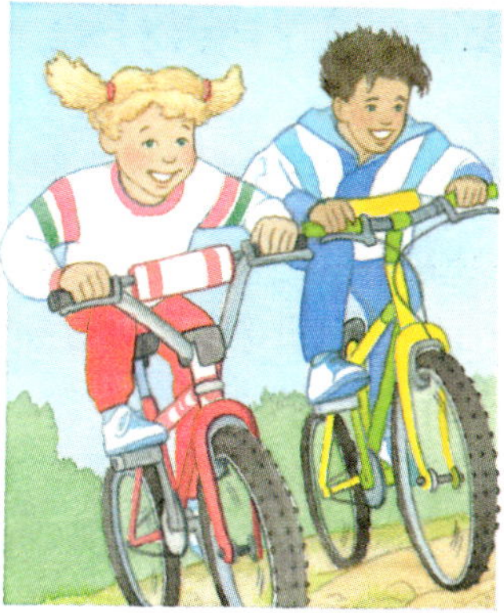

Carbohydrates supply energy to keep the body going.

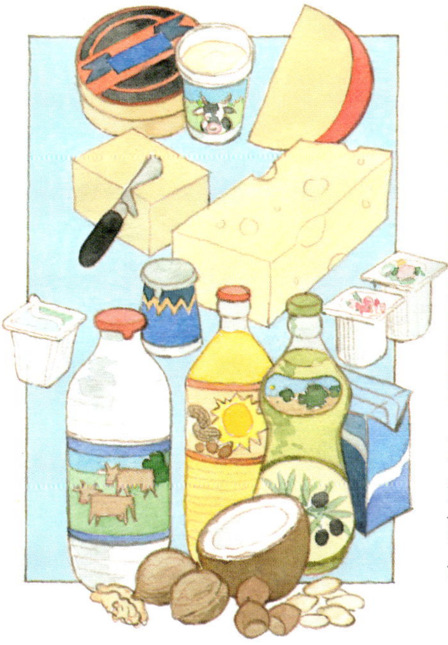

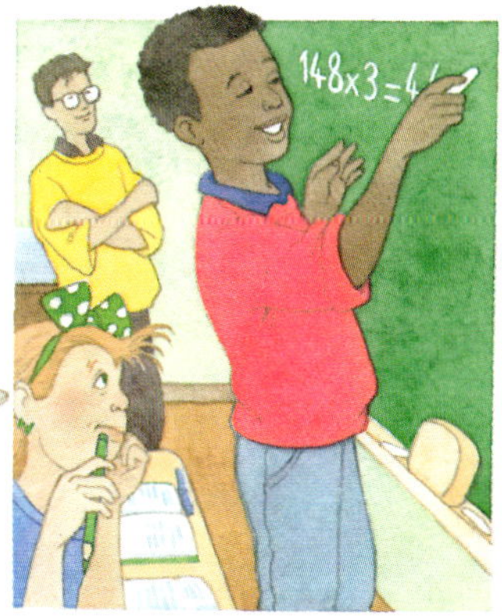

Fats store energy for the body to use, but we shouldn't eat too much fat.

☺ Vitamins

The body needs vitamins to work smoothly. These six vitamins are in our food.

VITAMIN A
for good eyesight and healthy skin.

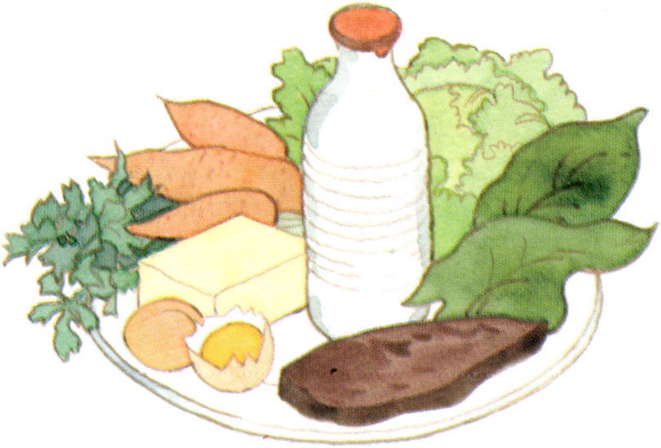

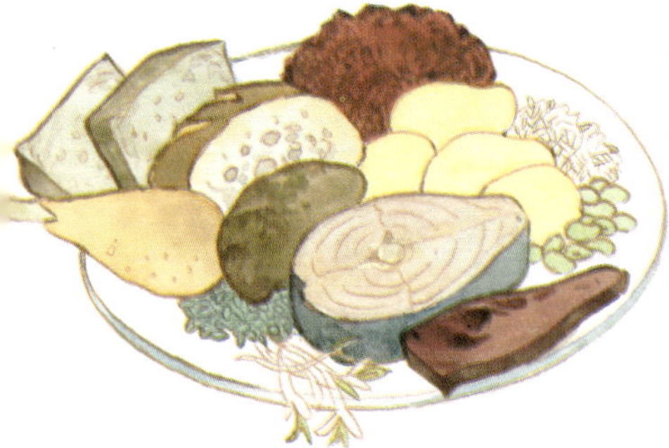

VITAMIN B
to help turn food into energy, and for healthy skin and nerves

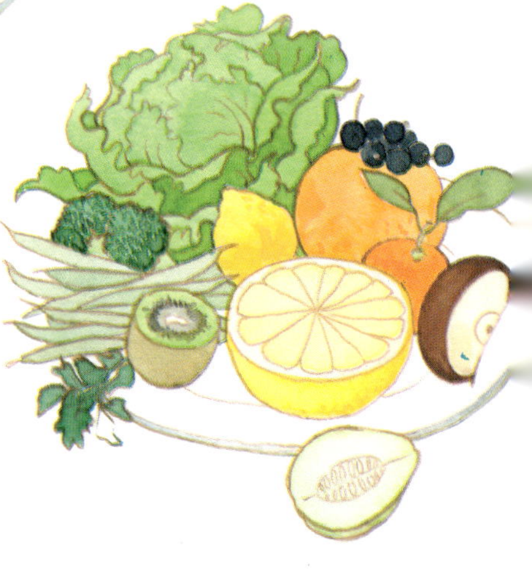

VITAMIN C
to help us recover from illness quickly, and to help wounds heal.

It is important to eat vitamins every day, because our bodies do not produce enough of them all.

VITAMIN D
to help us grow.

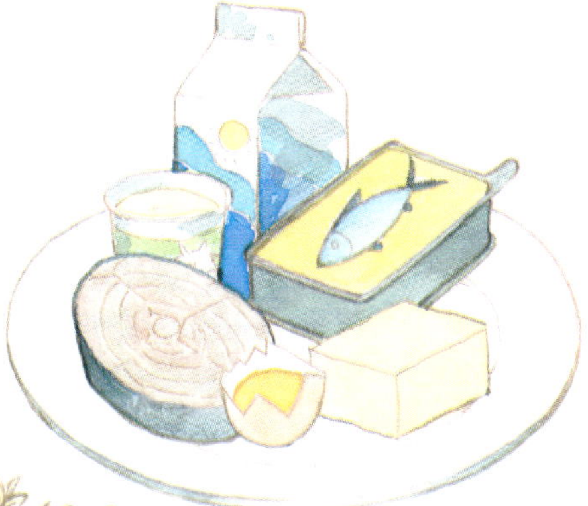

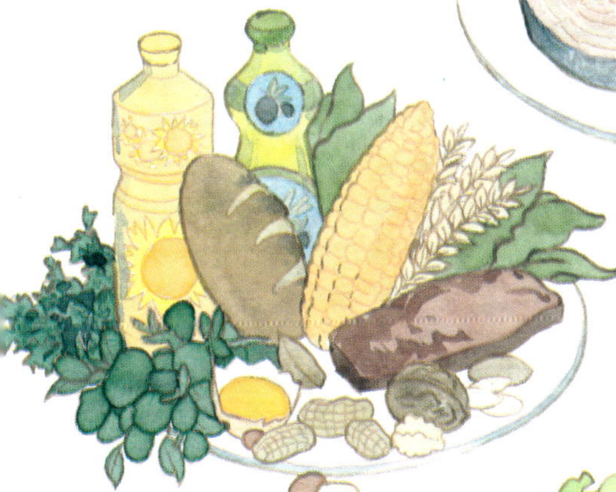

VITAMIN E
to help the body's cells stay strong.

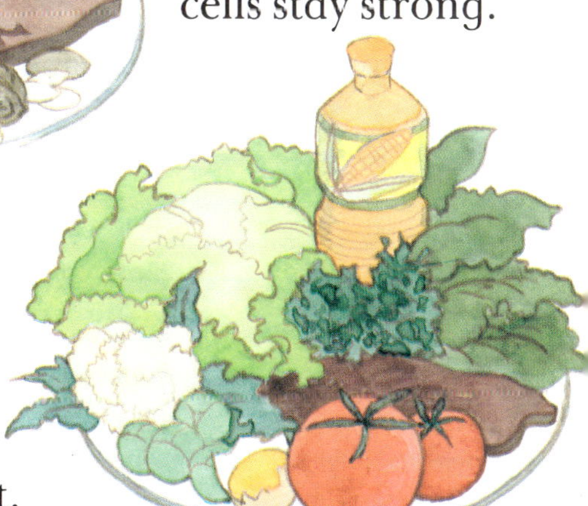

VITAMIN K
to help our blood clot, so that we don't bleed too much if we get a cut.

Keeping clean

Our skin gets dirty. It is important to wash every day, because soap and water help to get rid of any germs. It is also nice for other people if we are clean and smell fresh.

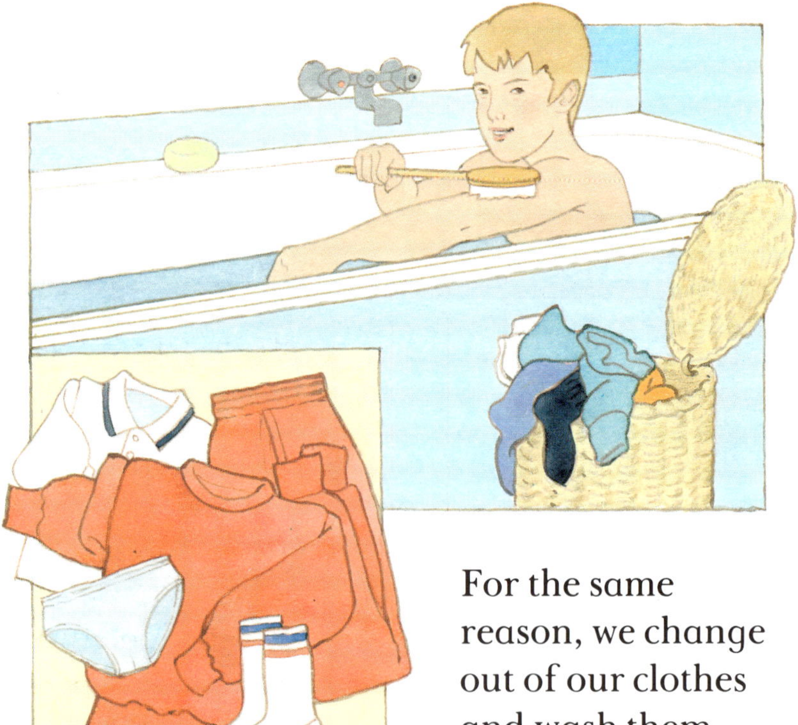

For the same reason, we change out of our clothes and wash them, and we put on clean clothes.

Washing your hair and your hands ...

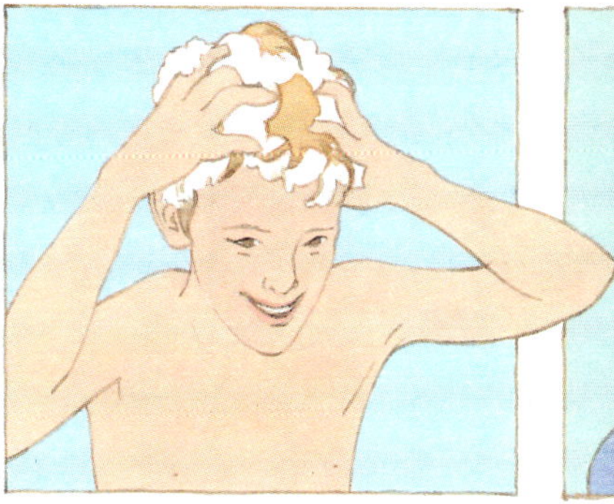

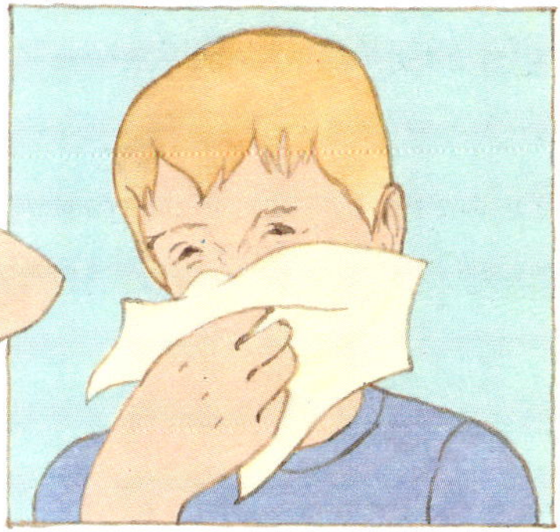

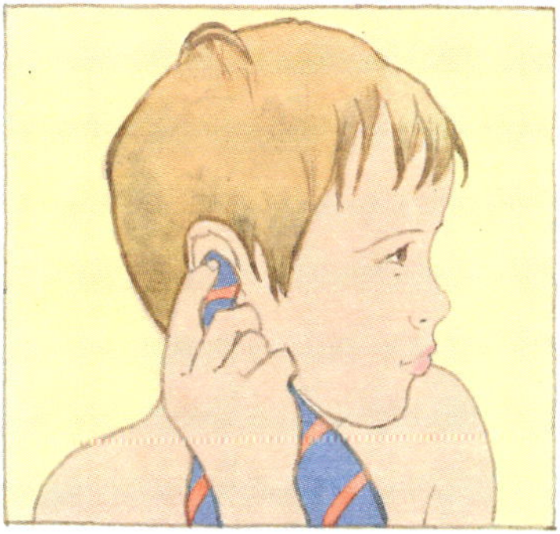

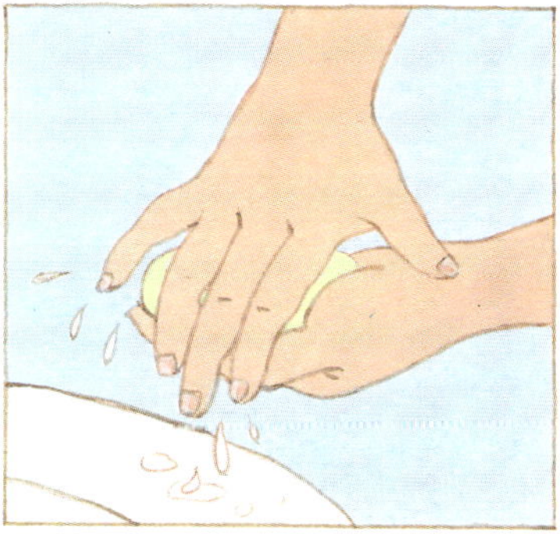

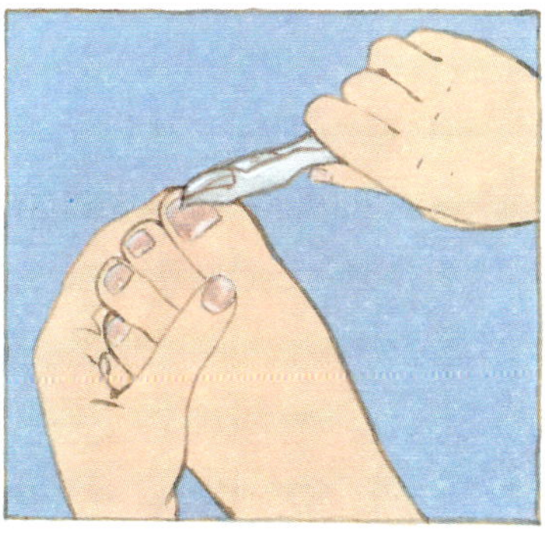

... cleaning your ears, cutting your nails, blowing your nose and brushing your teeth are all part of keeping clean.

☺ Dressing up

Clothes help the body to stay at the right temperature. We wear more clothes in cold weather than we do in hot weather. Clothes also protect our bodies. For example, we wear a helmet and pads when we play some sports.

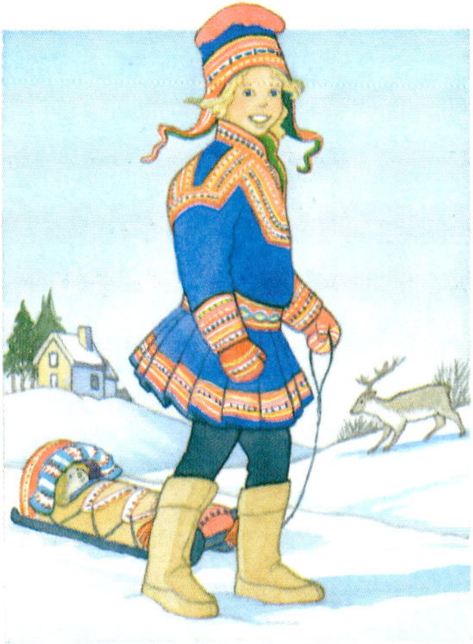

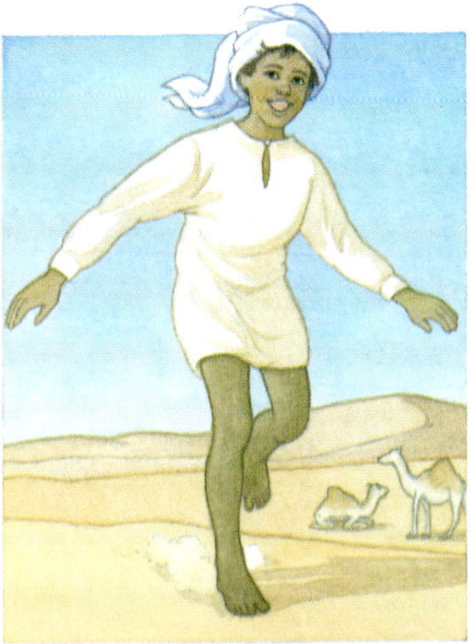

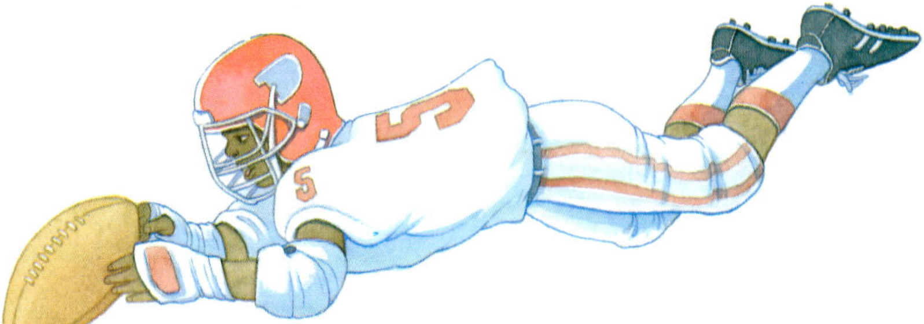

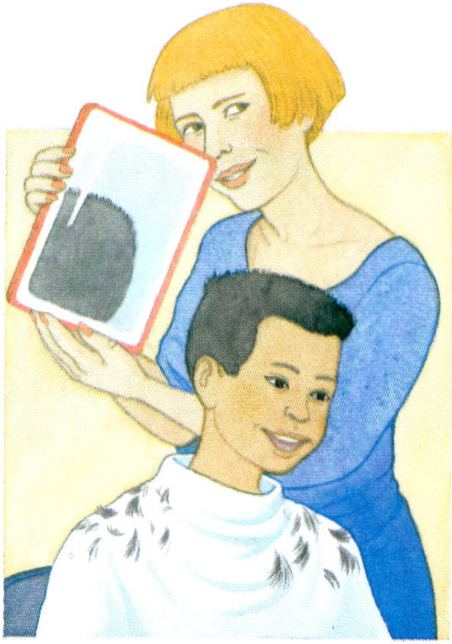

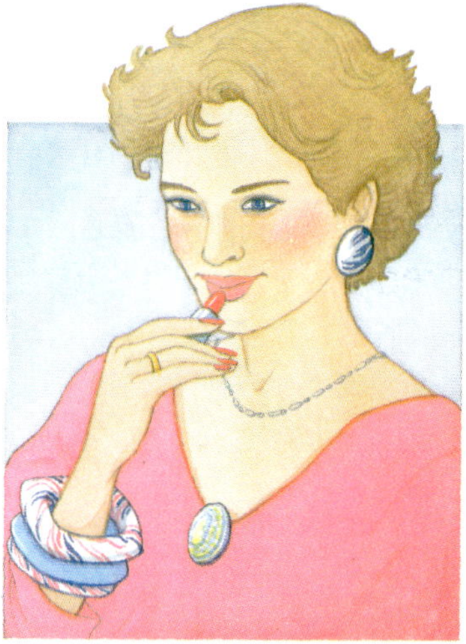

People dress up to make themselves look nice and feel good. We can choose a new hairstyle, wear some jewellery and put on some make-up, or wear a tie.

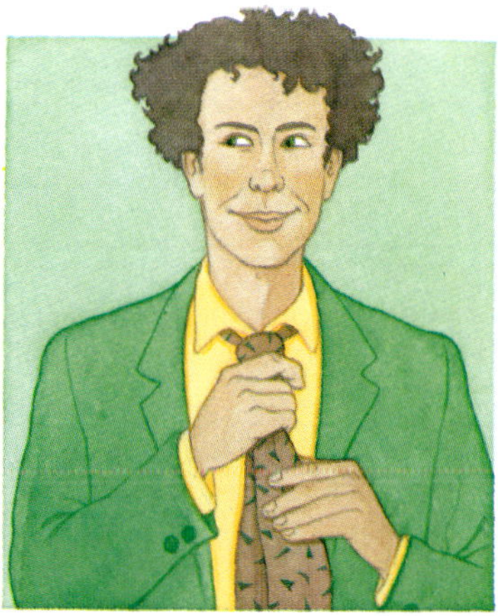

There are lots of styles and fashions to choose from. People dress up the way they like best.

☺ A happy life

Love and friendship and respect for each other make life happy for everyone.

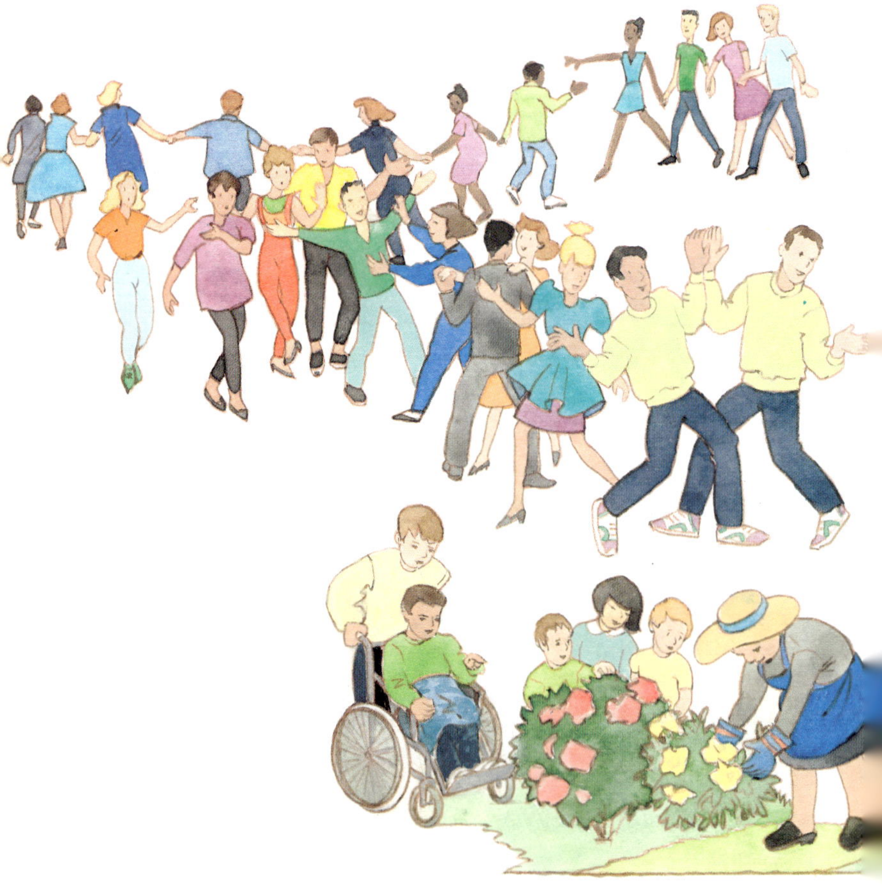

We express these feelings with our bodies – with a cuddle, a kiss, a hug, a smile, or an outstretched hand.

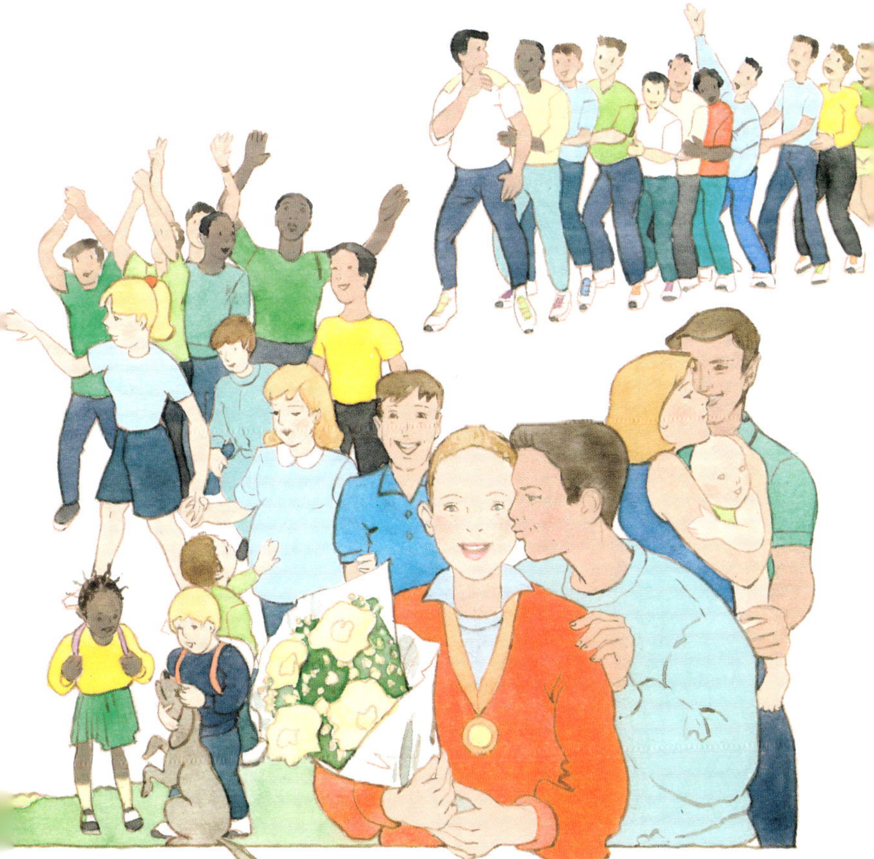

Funny phrases

If you want to describe a moment of great excitement or fear, you can say: "*My heart was in my mouth!*" Parts of the body are often used in phrases like this. Here are some more examples:

When you try to remember the right word, it's often *on the tip of your tongue.*

To put your foot in it means to make a blunder. But if things go wrong, just *keep your hair on* or stay cool!

The apple of your eye is your favourite person.

When something costs *an arm and a leg*, it is very expensive.

INDEX

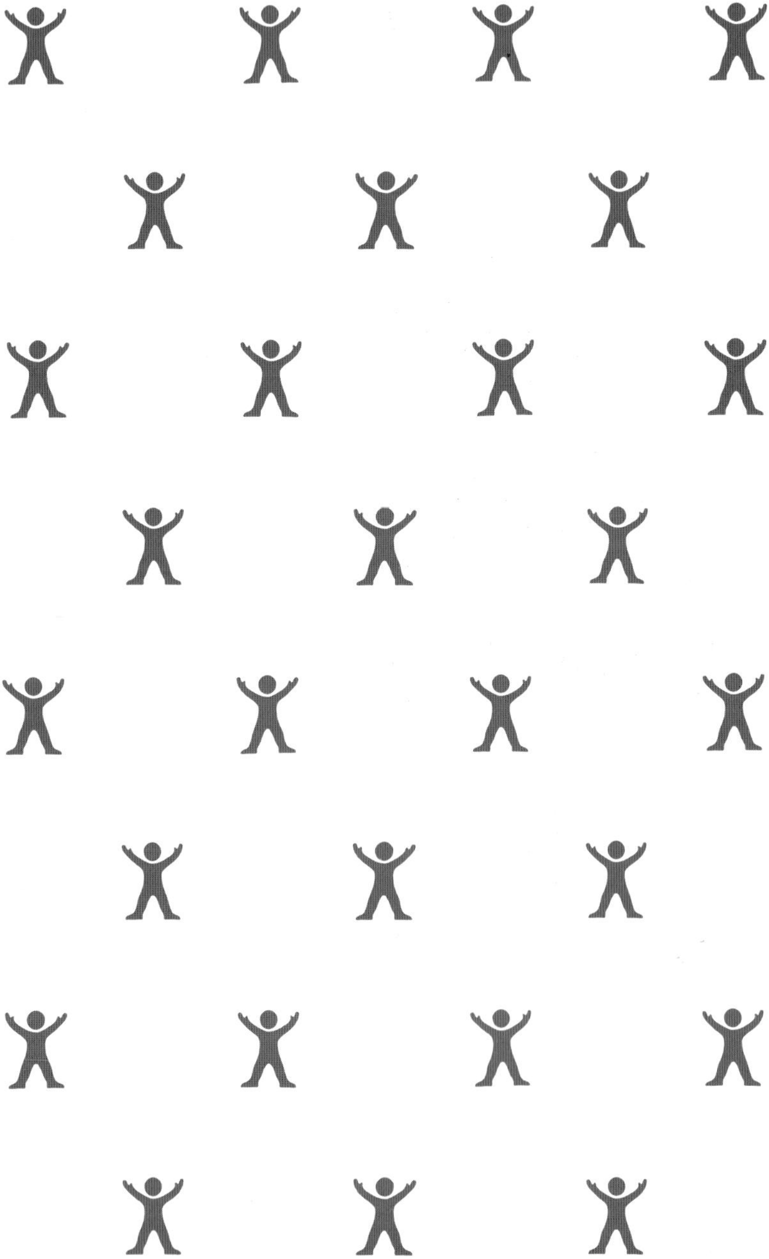

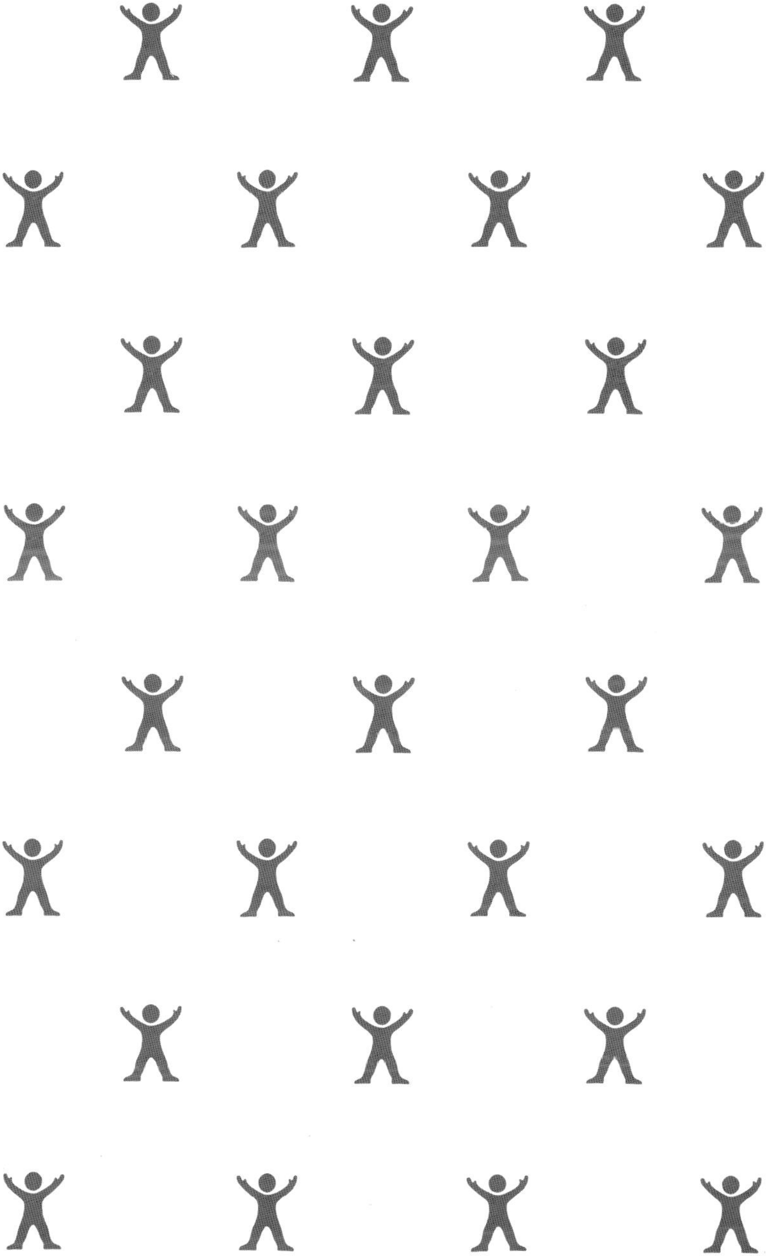